Neuro Care Revolution: Saving Money, Saving Lives

Neuro Care Revolution: Saving Money, Saving Lives

Shah

First Printing, 2024

Hold on to your hats, Horace! This journey's been longer and weirder than anyone could have imagined

Contents

1. Introduction

The prospects of an increasing proportion of the elderly population result in increased healthcare budgets. Eurostat expects the median age of European citizens to increase by 3.8 years by 2050, and the number of centenarians to raise to half a million by that date [69]. Inevitably, this aging will increase the prevalence of age-related disorders, such as neurodegenerative diseases [79, 126]. This is expected to raise costs for healthcare accordingly [68]. The problem of monitoring an increasing number of patients with age-related neurodegenerative disorders is aggravated by the fact that the amount of neurologists in Europe is far too low [56]. Hence, it is imperative to develop automated procedures that help diminishing costs while maintaining high-quality healthcare for elderly people. Cost containment can benefit from remote monitoring procedures using simple and inexpensive tests, both reducing the need of having patients to visit their neurologists in person, and enabling automated monitoring procedures.

An additional problem with neurodegenerative diseases is the nature of the current methods used to monitor their progress. For example, in the case of Parkinson's Disease (PD). PD is a common neurodegenerative disease, requiring constant monitoring to perform adjustments of pharmacological interventions, to assess risks, and to monitor its progress [200]. The clinical standard used till date to monitor its progress is the Unified Parkinson's Disease Rating Scale (UPDRS) [108]. When a neurologist evaluates the severity of, for example, the hand tremor of a PD patient using UPDRS, they are requested to observe the patients while they perform a series of manual tasks (e.g., opening and closing their fist). The neurologist is then tasked with evaluating tremor severity, on a zero (no problems) to four (unable to complete the task) scale, through visual observation. However, the criteria to grade a tremor as a one, two, or three is considerably ambiguous. Regular UPDRS assessment is usually accompanied by a home diary [121], which inevitably includes the subjective view of the patient. It is a well-documented fact that this subjectivity and ambiguity introduces sensitivity and reliability problems [243]. The risk of misdiagnosis and late diagnosis in PD is also commonly mentioned [212]. Furthermore, the relationship between PD and coexisting neurodegenerative diseases that present very similar symptoms, and how to effectively distinguish them, is not yet really understood [137].

A potential solution to this problem is to use health information technologies, in the form of sensors and classification techniques, which provide more objective assessment methods. These technologies are proven to increase the quality and cost-efficiency of medical care [41]. Sensors, unlike traditional assessment methods, can continuously collect rich, objective physiological data from users. The scientific community has already been aware of the potential role of these sensors for monitoring and diagnosis [192].

The use of sensors and classification techniques in health information technologies has led to the conception of clinical decision support systems. These systems are technological creations designed to support clinicians in decision-making tasks, by providing them with richer data as a basis for therapeutic options and decisions [225] (*Figure 1*). For example, these systems have been successfully implemented in early cancer detection [175] and post-operatory complication prediction [217].

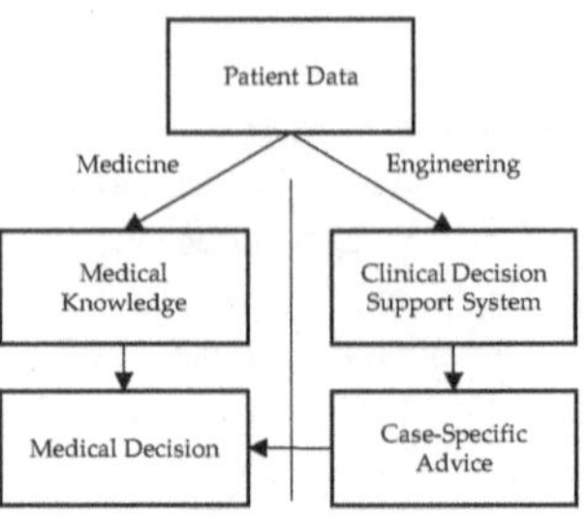

Figure 1: Role of a clinical decision support system

The success of clinical decision support systems depends on a number of factors other than predictive accuracy, such as minimizing user-provided data or involving caregivers in the development process [38]. This presents a twofold problem. On the one hand, it is important to collect as much relevant data as possible to maximize prediction accuracy. On the other hand, this should be done without being unnecessarily intrusive to the patient, particularly if the system is intended to be used by outpatients at home regularly. This means that data collection should occur in the background whenever feasible, and active participation, if needed, should be as engaging as possible.

1.1. Motivation for Exergame-based Clinical Decision Support Systems

To address the current limitations of clinical decision support systems, a reasonable possibility is to incorporate serious games into the formula [287]. Serious games are videogames with an additional goal beyond entertainment. For example, serious games that require and encourage users to perform physical exercise are called exergames. The use of exergame-based interventions in PD has already been successfully explored [92]. Recent randomized clinical trials have compared the outcome of using exergame-based rehabilitation with traditional rehabilitation, which is usually traditional physical exercise. Preliminary results indicate that when the exergames are specifically developed to address the physical needs of PD patients, results are at least as positive as with traditional rehabilitation. An additional advantage has also been observed: exergames also improve the patient's cognitive skills to an extent [235]. This is also reflected in previous research: physical rehabilitation has been observed to improve cognition in PD patients [127], and cognitive training has been observed to improve physical symptoms [333]. As such, exergames seem to be an ideal method to implement this combination of cognitive and physical rehabilitation, also known as dual-tasking [261].

Although exergame-based interventions seem to be ideal for PD patients, the potential for a clinical decision support system to gather data from these exergames to monitor the progress of PD is yet to be explored. Usually, the effectiveness of exergame-based interventions is measured by traditional and potentially subjective PD assessment methods. However, the potential for clinical decision support systems to monitor PD symptoms has been analyzed by different researchers [50, 211, 318, 334]. For this reason, designing clinical decision support systems that collect data from these exergame-based interventions, and using them to monitor the patients, is a very promising approach. By using an exergame-based clinical decision support system, data could be collected in the background while the user is playing, providing the caregiver with meaningful clinical information. The exergame could add the necessary attractiveness to trigger and motivate the user into using the system as often as the data collection procedure requires, without the need for cueing users to do so. Similar approaches have been suggested in the past, but have not yet been explored in detail [171, 292]. Based on this situation, we have defined the following research gap that this book aims to cover:

Research gap. *The feasibility of developing exergame-based clinical decision support systems that can objectively monitor the symptoms of chronic diseases, as well as the potential benefit of these systems for the patients, is yet to be explored.* To address this gap, this book proposes an abstract approach for a clinical decision support system used to monitor a chronic disease that uses exergames for data acquisition. The goal of this book is also to implement this model with the example of PD and validate the outcomes of this implementation in comparison with standard PD clinical outcomes.

1.2. Research Challenges

To explore this research gap, we aim at developing a model for an exergame-based clinical decision support system. We identify the following challenges that influence the design and potential success of this system.

Challenge: *Identifying, conceiving, and implementing viable sensors that can be used both as control devices for exergames and to provide clinically meaningful data.* Designing a sensor-based environment that can be used to monitor a certain symptom of a chronic disease is a task that must be performed on a case-by-case basis. First, it is necessary to understand the nature of the symptom, how it physically manifests, and whether this manifestation can be objectively measured with a sensor. If this is possible, the sensor chosen (or designed) to monitor this symptom must also function as a control device to operate an exergame. We chose to focus this book on PD because it is the second most common neurodegenerative disease after Alzheimer's disease [183], and presents well-known and well-identified physical symptoms. In addition, as discussed, its current assessment standards show subjectivity and reliability problems [243]. The most important physical symptoms caused by PD are also known as "cardinal signs." These cardinal signs are resting tremor, rigidity, bradykinesia (slowness of movement), and postural instability (balance affection, leading to falls) [200]. In parallel to physical symptoms, PD also presents a progressive cognitive degeneration [226]. In both cases, these symptoms present significant interindividual variability [200]. For this book, we chose to focus on two of these cardinal signs: balance and hand tremor. We chose these two symptoms in agreement with medical partners because they can be measured with sensors, they have no correlation among themselves (other than being symptoms of PD) and are measurable with the minimal personal information possible.

Challenge: *Designing dual-tasking exergames that permit the acquisition of clinically meaningful data while being attractive to the target population.* Once a viable symptom-sensor combination has been identified, an exergame must be designed around the data acquisition process. If this data acquisition requires active participation (e.g., performing a certain movement in a certain way), the exergame must incorporate this participation as part of its control pattern. In addition, the exergame must offer attractiveness and engagement, using the data to adapt the difficulty and ensuring that patients are willing to use the system over a long period and thus clinically meaningful data can be collected in this manner.

1.3. Research Goals

The main objective of this book is to conceive, design and implement an exergame-based clinical decision support system capable of assessing the risk of falling and the severity of hand tremors of PD patients. We divide this objective into two main research goals, and two secondary research goals:

Research Goal 1. *Design an exergame-based clinical decision support system capable of assessing the risk of falling.* To achieve this goal, we employ an array of synchronized Wii Balance Boards. This system, called Extended Balance Board, allows us to evaluate balance while standing and walking [88]. We implement classification features used to determine potential instability, based on information about the player's center of mass. We also present PDDanceCity [91], a dual-tasking exergame designed to train balance and cognition, that drives this system. Finally, we evaluate the capability of this system to predict if a player has an increased risk of falling based on the result of the so-called 30-Second Sit to Stand Test [20]. The materials and methods developed to achieve this goal are described in *Chapter 5.* We also implemented an approach alternative to the Extended Balance Board in the section *Alternative Balance Assessment System* [168] for comparison. The implementation of this system represents the proof of concept of the model presented in this book to monitor the risk of falling.

Research Goal 2. *Design an exergame-based clinical decision support system capable of assessing hand tremors.* We achieve this goal by using Leap Motion sensors. First, we develop a data acquisition and signal processing framework capable of extracting clinically meaningful data from a series of hand movements similar to the ones performed in the UPDRS test. We call this framework Parkinson Assessment with Leap Motion (PALM) [99]. We also design a dual-tasking exergame based on hand movements similar to those of the UPDRS test, entitled PDPuzzleTable, which also includes cognitive exercises and thus dual-tasking [93]. Finally, we evaluate the system in its capability to correctly discriminate PD patients from healthy controls. We chose the Leap Motion sensor because of its non-invasive nature since users do not have to wear any device on themselves. However, there are numerous other potential approaches to objectively assess hand tremors. These approaches are described in the section *Assessing Resting Tremor* and *Appendix B.* The implementation of this system represents the proof of concept of the model presented in this book to monitor hand tremors.

Secondary Goal 1. *Explore the possibility of monitoring additional relevant PD symptoms continuously as part of the developed systems.* We consider the possibility of implementing the monitoring of two additional relevant PD symptoms into the developed systems: (1) heart-rate changes and (2) blink-rate alterations. We chose these two symptoms because they can be monitored non-invasively and as part of the concept presented in *Chapter 4,* and are also relevant to PD as described in *Chapter 3.* For this purpose, data acquisition should occur in the background without active participation from the patient whenever possible. We present two novel non-invasive biosignal acquisition algorithms in *Chapter 7.* The accuracy of these algorithms has also been evaluated. However, their potential use in PD would require acquiring data from the users on a long-term basis (years), and as such, they are not presented as one of the main components of this book.

Secondary Goal 2. *Explore alternative game-based interventions in PD other than exergames.* We also study the possibility of using two alternative game-based interventions in PD other than exergames: Virtual

Reality (VR), and Brain-Computer Interfaces (BCI). Our initial research and preliminary results did not elicit designing exergames with these approaches. The results of our analysis are included in *Chapter 8*.

1.4. Structure of the book

This book is structured in nine chapters. All chapters include a brief summary of the content at the beginning. The section *Previously Published Material* describes the scientific publications that comprise the content of this book, and the contributions of the author to these publications. *Chapter 1, Introduction,* describes the motivation behind this book and its research challenges and goals. *Chapter 2, Foundations,* provides a description of the background for this research: serious games, telemedicine, and clinical decision support systems. A description of PD and UPDRS is included in *Appendix A. Chapter 3, Related Work,* describes the summarized results of two systematic reviews on related work that comprise our requirement analysis, while further details of these reviews are provided in *Appendix B* and *Appendix C. Chapter 4, Model for an Exergame-based Clinical Decision Support System,* presents our formalized model to achieve the goals of this book, with additional design details included in *Appendix D.* This model is then implemented for two different scenarios in *Chapter 5, Design of an Exergame-based Clinical Decision Support System to Assess Balance* and *Chapter 6, Design of an Exergame-based Clinical Decision Support System to Assess Tremor.* Additional experimental details for these two implementations are provided in *Appendix E* and *Appendix F.* This implementation is complemented by two biosignal acquisition algorithms presented in *Chapter 7, Heart-rate Estimation Algorithm* and *Blink-rate Estimation Algorithm.* We discuss two alternative game based approaches to exergames in *Chapter 8, Brain-Computer Interfaces* and *Virtual Reality.* Further experimental details for these two chapters are included in *Appendix G* and *Appendix H.* A summary, including an outlook and potential future work, is presented in *Chapter 9, Summary, Conclusions and Future Work.* The two final appendices are *Appendix I, List of Acronyms,* and *Appendix J, Supervised Student Theses.* This book also includes a list of *Publications* of the author and his *Curriculum Vitae.*

2. Foundations

In this chapter, we present a brief background to the topics that comprise the design of exergame-based clinical decision support systems as motivated in *Chapter 1*. We start with an introduction into serious games and exergames, their current challenges, and fields of research. This is followed by a definition of the concept of remote patient monitoring. A general description of clinical decision support systems follows. A medical description of PD, its symptoms, and its assessment methods can be consulted in *Appendix A*.

2.1. Serious Games and Exergames

Serious games are digital interactive applications created with a main purpose beyond entertainment, called its "characterizing goal." This implies that serious games are intended both to be entertaining and to fulfil another goal, such as a learning effect or a behavioral change in nutritional habits [61]. In particular, serious games with the characterizing goal of improving physical health are called exertion games or, for short, exergames [61] (*Figure* 2).

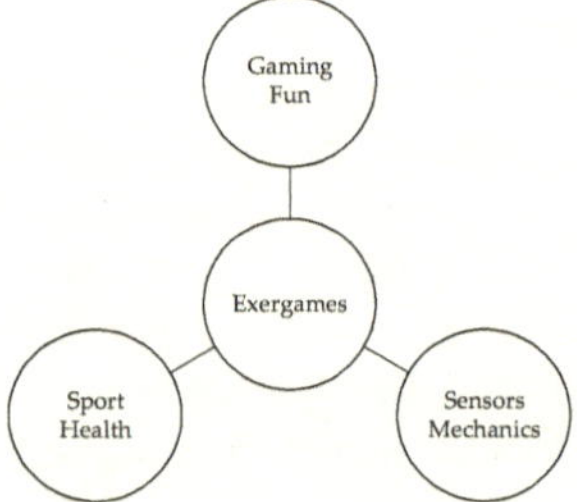

Figure 2: Contributing elements in the field of exergames, derived from [120]

Serious games provide an approach that is of interest in a broad spectrum of application sectors, ranging from education [213], game-based learning [336], and particularly its collaborative aspects [267], to social awareness (energy, climate, security, etc.) or health. The healthcare arena is a main application domain of serious games [61]. For example, Göbel et al. [106] explored the role serious games play in interaction techniques, sensor-based monitoring systems, and the acquisition of biosignals. In their opinion, these vital signs and sensor data can be directly employed in personalized exergames, following the Monitoring, Analysis, Planning and Execution Loop [10]. Gameplay and the vital status of users are recorded, analyzed and interpreted, and the game is adapted accordingly. This becomes particularly useful when the skills and characteristics of users are expected to have significant interindividual variability, as is the case with PD. Here, adaptive exergames allow dynamic difficulty adaptation both for cognitive and physical exercises in PD rehabilitation programs.

In recent years, a number of challenges have been identified and addressed in the field of serious games in general and adaptive exergaming in particular [105]. Researchers focus on the importance of adaptation, particularly if the target population has disabilities [339]. The importance of creating pervasive interventions [64], particularly how to improve adherence with data-based approaches to trigger users at the right moment, is explored in the Ph.D. book of Dutz [63], following the basic principles of Fogg [81]. The importance of the impact of exergame-based interventions, as well as the perceptions users have of this impact, has also been identified as a relevant factor [70]. Concerning data analysis, multimodal analytics methods should be applied to adaptive exergames, since different streams of data of a very diverse nature (i.e. video, audio, sensor data and biosignals) are to be expected, as discussed in Shoukry et al. [284].

In the present book, we incorporate these recent advances by ensuring that our exergames are adapted to the individual characteristics of our users. We also ensure that our exergames offer varying degrees of physical and cognitive difficulty, which can be adjusted based on game performance as measured by data extracted from the game itself.

2.2. Remote Patient Monitoring and Telemedicine

Broadly, telemedicine is defined as the use of communication technology to provide healthcare remotely [128]. This may refer to the use of remote audio or video communications, or other technological means, to perform physician consultations, diagnose potential diseases (screening), or monitor existing ones (patient monitoring). A simple sensor-based telemedicine system can consist, for example, of a device that measures heart-rate, blood pressure or blood glucose levels, and sends these to a physician or caregiver continuously. The main advantage of these systems is that they provide clinically meaningful information with a frequency that is unachievable with a traditional approach (i.e. weekly clinician visits). A subset of particular interest in remote patient monitoring is the use of mobile technologies, such as smartphones. This is commonly defined as mobile health or mHealth [97, 208]. mHealth presents the additional advantage of combining the sensors and communication device in a single, ubiquitous system. Almost half of the worldwide population owns a smartphone [233, 249], which means there are 3.5 billion potential remote patient monitoring devices at this moment. The interest of patients in using telemedicine is also growing. For example, Teladoc, an industry leader in telemedicine, regularly reports a yearly increase in patient visits above 70 percent [310], which further increased to 90 percent in the midst of the COVID-19 pandemic [311].

The main research areas in telemedicine, other than practical implementations, are reliability and privacy. The introduction of blockchain [344], and of 5G and edge computing [134], are potential solutions to these problems. Sensor fusion and data quality assessment techniques [216] are also relevant. The onset of COVID-19 and stay-at-home orders have accentuated the need for implementing functional telemedicine strategies [17, 128, 236, 344].

In the specific example of PD, many assessment tests can be administered remotely, and could be significantly improved by technical means. In fact, studies exploring the feasibility of including telemedicine as part of PD monitoring indicate substantial interest, particularly for early PD and patients with long commutes [259]. The PDExergames project [319], in the framework of which many of the methods of this book have been elaborated, considers PD as a potential application scenario for exergame-based remote patient monitoring.

2.3. Clinical Decision Support Systems

A clinical decision support system is a technical tool that provides medical practitioners with an additional stream of information on which to base clinical decisions [28]. Clinical decision support systems provide numerous advantages: they can increase the quality and efficiency of health care and reduce the occurrence of errors [28]. Broadly, a clinical decision support system usually consists of two elements. The first element is a medical data source, for example a patient who has recently received major surgery. From this medical data source, technical data are derived. Following this example, vital signs such as heart-rate, heart-rate variability, blood pressure, and blood oxygen saturation, may be collected. These technical data are then processed into features, that is, curated data that contain information pertinent to the classification problem. The features are then employed by the second element: a classifier algorithm (e.g., a neural network). The output of this classifier, whose accuracy depends on the technical data, is then translated into clinically relevant information. Continuing this example, this information could provide valuable knowledge about the potential risk the patient has of developing post operatory complications [217] (*Figure* 3).

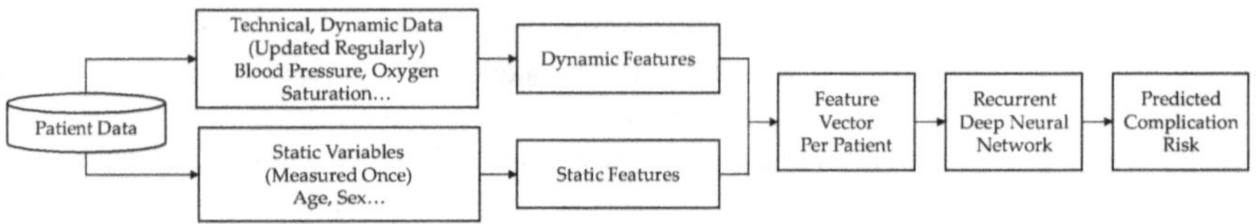

Figure 3: Model of a clinical decision support system, presented in [217]

From a medical perspective, the taxonomy of clinical decision support systems can be determined by their setting. Different systems are used for screening, diagnosis, treatment, drug dosing, test ordering, chronic disease management and health related behaviors. According to this taxonomy, most clinical decision support systems are used for either screening, drug dosing, or chronic disease management, the latter of which is the case in this book [225].

From a technical perspective, clinical decision support systems represent the use of novel computer science and electrical engineering methods in health information technology. These methods include natural language processing, outlier detection, other classification algorithms, sensor technologies, and novel signal processing techniques. Clinical decision support systems contribute to diminish paper medical records, speed up diagnostic procedures, and help sift vast amounts of information that would otherwise be incomprehensible [225]. This provides new medical technology methods which improve, refine or outperform the previous ones. In this sense, clinical decision support systems are, as described in [225], at the heart of a "learning healthcare system." Novel clinical decision support systems improve how professionals care for patients, these improvements are recorded, and new treatment and diagnosis standards are established. Based on these results, improved medical outcomes set a new scenario in which to implement novel clinical decision support systems, thus continuing the cycle.

The main challenge clinical decision support systems face is their slow implementation. In [38], Castillo et al. discuss numerous factors that may be taken into consideration when addressing this challenge. In this book, we involve caregivers in the design process and aim to reduce user-entered data to a minimum. In addition, we aim to provide further evidence that clinical decision support systems are effective in providing objective conclusions that highly correlate with traditional assessment scales and clinical standards.

3. Related Work

Having presented an overview of the foundations for this book in *Chapter 2*, in this chapter we study recent publications related to this book. Related work primarily concerns two domains: sensor-based monitoring of PD symptoms, and exergame-based PD interventions. We conducted systematic reviews in both areas. In the first section, we focus on the symptoms related to the goals of this book: balance and gait, hand tremors, and the effect of bradykinesia in hand dexterity. We also discuss other symptoms such as blink-rate and heart-rate affections, which could potentially be monitored with the system presented in this book. This work was performed partly as student theses [114, 291]. Numerous studies indicate the possibility of monitoring many symptoms of PD with technical, objective means. This is particularly the case with balance and resting hand tremor. The Leap Motion sensor has great potential for this specific purpose. *Appendix B* includes further details of this review. In the second section, we analyze recent studies on exergame-based interventions in PD with the goal of rehabilitation. We identified several clinical trials, which elicited a meta-analysis [187] of their results. This work was published as an article in the Journal of Neuroengineering and Rehabilitation [92]. These clinical trials have proven the feasibility of exergame-based PD rehabilitation. Preliminary results show this rehabilitation to be as effective as traditional rehabilitation. However, limited sample sizes suggest that further, more comprehensive trials are required. Studies indicate the importance of task specificity (developing exergames targeted towards the cognitive and physical domains of PD) and using standard outcomes, such as the UPDRS. Details of this meta-analysis are provided in *Appendix C*. This section also discusses alternative approaches to exergames that we explored. We developed two systems using these alternatives, described in *Appendix H*.

3.1. Sensor-based Approaches to Monitor Symptoms of Parkinson's Disease

PD patients monitor the evolution of their symptoms with the help of a diary of motor symptoms [258]. Though helpful, this diary may lack sensitivity and objectivity. In recent years, numerous studies aiming towards objective, sensor-based alternatives have been produced. To analyze related work in this area, we performed a systematic review search for studies published in the PubMed database, from January 1, 2010 to June 29, 2017 (the date of the last search). We conducted our analysis using the final search string: *"Sensor* OR Wearable* AND Parkinson*."* An asterisk represents all words that contain the character, regardless of termination.

This search yielded 3062 results at the last query. Inclusion criteria were articles concerning a sensor-based approach to monitor a motor PD symptom. The exclusion criterion was articles not including an evaluation on PD patients attempting to predict a clinical outcome (2886 exclusions). This review was conducted in accordance with the Preferred Reporting Items for Systematic Reviews and Meta-Analyses (PRISMA) guidelines [221]. These criteria yielded 156 articles. We selected the articles in regard to their measurement approach and performance. The survey was completed by analyzing publications referenced by those articles. After conducting this review and while implementing our approach, we identified and included 20 additional publications. We found a number of studies discussing the use of the Leap Motion sensor to monitor tremors and bradykinesia, especially from 2018 onwards. The complete results of this systematic review are provided in *Appendix B*. We summarize the main outcomes of this review for each symptom as follows.

Assessing Balance and Gait

PD affects both balance and gait in different ways. The main risk postural imbalance poses for PD patients is an increased risk of falling. Recent studies suggest that more than half of PD patients experience falls, and one fourth will fracture their hip due to falling. Higher UPDRS scores are main predictors for this risk. A decay in the effectiveness of levodopa, a dopamine replacement drug for PD treatment [86], also plays a role. Patients with mostly nondopaminergic symptoms do not seem to experience this risk [12]. This means that PD patients on levodopa are at increased risk of falling, and this risk increases as the disease advances. Thus, falls are relevant to monitor the state of PD patients, especially those with advanced PD in nursing homes. Both wearables and smartphone applications capable of detecting falls are currently available, non-invasively detecting falls with high accuracy [334]. The Microsoft Kinect sensor has also been identified as a potential monitoring solution [248, 297, 298, 307] as well as a fall detection system [301].

The possibility of using pressure plates, such as the Wii Balance Board, to estimate fall risk has also been identified [305]. Since these plates can be used to control exergames, these studies are closely related to this book. The Wii Balance Board has been shown to accurately distinguish between elderly people who fell in the past and others who did not based on center of pressure data [215]. Researchers also report that there are differences in the way users with increased risk of falling interact with the Wii Balance Board [342]. These studies are summarized in *Table 2*.

Reference	N	Cohort	Features	Goal	Results
Mertes et al. [215]	12	Healthy elderly	Center of pressure data	Classify between fallers and non-fallers	76.6% Classification accuracy using Support Vector Machines
Yamada et al. [342]	45	Healthy elderly	Wii Fit Game scores (Basic Step and Ski Slalom)	Correlate game performance with fall history and find differences in fallers	Significant differences ($p<.001$) and moderate correlations ($r=0.69$)

Table 2: Recent studies predicting balance skills with Wii Balance Board data

Another gait affection in PD is freeze of gait. It is a sudden but temporary halt of the patient's gait despite an intention to walk that affects approximately 50% of PD patients, especially men and those with advanced PD. It depends on the environment, and is thus difficult to reproduce in laboratory conditions. Freeze of gait severely impairs quality of life and also causes falls. These gait alterations seem to be related to cognitive deterioration [103], but are dopaminergic in nature and therefore normally, but not exclusively, appear during OFF periods (periods where levodopa is not working). Freeze of gait episodes can be detected by measuring foot ground reaction or ankle acceleration. In this second case, an episode can be detected if the spectral density in the 3-8 Hz band outranges a certain threshold. This is of particular interest, since it is the same frequency band that PD tremor is present at, as described in the section *Assessing Resting Tremor*. Recent studies predict episodes of freezing of gait using this method [16, 211]. However, they mention that this symptom shows significant interindividual differences. The possibility of using commercial gait sensors, such as gait analysis running wearables, is as yet unexplored. In *Chapter 5*, we study the possibility of using an array of Wii Balance Boards to this end.

Once detected, possible solutions to reduce the impact of freeze of gait have been studied, including rhythmic or musical cues. Visual or somatosensory cues do not seem to produce any improvement [16]. The best cue seems to be a rhythmical metronome ticking sound with a rate slightly higher than the patient's usual pace. In a limited study with 10 PD patients, users of such a system subjectively reported less and shorter episodes, and indicated that such a device would improve their quality of life. The users were annoyed when the cueing system activated itself too frequently, while users with low sensitivity requested more frequent activations. However, no field study has been performed so far confirming the effectiveness of such a system in reducing symptoms [16]. In fact, no studies have shown that such a system reduces the frequency or duration of freezing of gait episodes. Nevertheless, such a system could potentially be implemented in an exergame-based scenario.

Assessing Resting Tremor

Parkinsonian tremor is a resting, pill-rolling movement. It is typically present in the 3-7 Hz frequency range, has an amplitude higher than 0.1 mV, and a burst duration of 50 to 150 ms [219]. This tremor can be measured by placing a smartphone in the dorsum of the hand or using an armband. A detailed list of recent approaches towards accurately measuring tremors using smartphones and wearables is provided in *Appendix B.*

Diseases different than PD also cause hand tremors. Differences in the nature of parkinsonian and, for example, essential tremor, would benefit from technology-based differentiation to reduce the misdiagnosis ratio. This can be done by evaluating data extracted from physical exercises or with electromyography [254]. Recent studies show that measuring tremor using an accelerometer for 60 seconds can be used to distinguish essential from parkinsonian tremor with an accuracy of over 90% [341]. This accuracy can be increased by recording tasks such as arm and hand movements [312].

Some technical designs also suggest the possibility of analyzing tremor non-invasively by using a hand control computer input device [117]. This would not require the user to wear the device. There are several options, such as glove-based solutions or infrared cameras. Although glove-based optoelectronic systems are believed to be more accurate [75], there are commercial off-the-shelf infrared cameras such as the Leap Motion sensor, which are more cost-effective [182, 245]. Using the Leap Motion sensor to monitor tremors and control exergames has shown promising results. The sensor is capable of detecting hand tremors [14, 42] and gestures [102]. Authors report increases in compliance and immersion when using the Leap Motion sensor in comparison to other therapies [9, 102]. Other studies indicate the potential of using the Leap Motion sensor to digitalize standard hand dexterity assessment tests [227]. However, the authors also indicate the importance of keeping the recording periods short [238].

The Leap Motion sensor can accurately measure low-frequency, high-amplitude tremors [164]. Concerning feature extraction, detecting halts and alterations in speed and acceleration are important factors [144, 277]. This is possible by using standard analysis features such as peak detection, analysis of averages, standard deviations, and amplitudes [42]. We identified a number of recent studies using the Leap Motion sensor to classify PD patients and controls and to estimate the severity of tremors, which is closely related to the goal of this book. A summary of these studies is presented in *Table 3*.

Preliminary results show high accuracy when using the Leap Motion sensor to classify PD patients and controls.

Reference	Device	N	Features	Goal	Classifier	Results (accuracy, sensitivity, specificity)
Johnson [139]	Leap Motion	30	Time- and frequency-domain features	Classify PD/Controls	Support Vector Machine	0.85,0.75,0.95
Butt et al. [30] (results are not separated between tremor and bradykinesia)	Leap Motion	28	Time- and frequency-domain features	Classify PD/Controls	Support Vector Machine	0.82,0.76,0.87
Vivar-Estudillo et al. [330]	Leap Motion	40	Statistical features	Classify PD/Controls	Bagged Tree	0.99,0.98,0.99
Lugo et al. [202]	Leap Motion	33	Time-domain, statistical and entropy features	Predict UPDRS III scores	Not specified	0.76,1.00,0.57
Kostikis [173]	Smartphone	25	Time-domain features	Predict UPDRS-III scores	Random Forest	0.90,0.82,0.90
Manzanera [209]	Accelerometer	14	Frequency-domain features	Detect tremor episodes	Welch	0.98,0.69,0.98

Table 3: Recent studies on Leap Motion sensor-based tremor assessment. A smartphone and conventional accelerometer approach are provided for comparison

Bradykinesia and dyskinesia

Bradykinesia (slowness of movement) and dyskinesias (uncontrolled movements) are very characteristic symptoms of PD. Shorter steps, feet dragging and slower movements when performing daily living activities are all part of bradykinesia. In [258], the authors used wrist and ankle motion sensors to monitor bradykinesia and dyskinesia to identify ON and OFF periods. The collected metrics agreed with blind clinician ratings, and their estimations correlated well with UPDRS scores (r=0.81). This approach was further improved in [130].

Bradykinesia also affects hand dexterity. The UPDRS test includes three tasks designed for evaluating this effect (see *Universal Parkinson's Disease Rating Scale*). We identified four studies that study the possibility of using the Leap Motion sensor to assess hand-dexterity, presented in *Table 4*. Based on these findings, we conclude that combining tremor and bradykinesia assessment should provide very accurate results when attempting to classify PD patients and controls. Recent studies indicate that speed-related features provide the most relevant information. However, attempting to predict task-specific UPDRS scores remains a challenging issue.

Reference	N	UPDRS Task	Leap Motion features	Goal	Result
Çakmak et al. [31]	24	Finger tapping	Local minima and maxima of the distances between thumb and index finger	Correlate features and UPDRS scores	Speed features provide best predictions, moderately accurate results (r=0.56)
Lee et al. [185]	8	Finger tapping, fist closing, pronation-supination	Angular displacement of the palm, median cosine angle between palm and intermediate phalanges, Euclidean distance between thumb and index finger	Correlate features and UPDRS scores	Speed features provide best predictions, strong correlations (r=0.86) between chosen features and neurologist assessment
Butt et al. [30] (results are not separated between tremor and bradykinesia)	28	Finger tapping, fist closing, pronation-supination	Palm angle, fingertip distance, fingertip velocity, frequency-domain features	Correlate features and UPDRS scores	Low correlations, but large effect sizes between healthy and controls for pronation-supination task (cohen's d=1.3)
Ferraris et al. [74]	57	Finger tapping, fist closing, pronation-supination	Time and frequency-domain features	Classify PD and controls Predict UPDRS scores	PD/control classification accuracy 98.97%, prediction of task-specific score accuracy of 76.71% for tapping, 66.21% for opening, 58.87% for pronation-supination

Table 4: Recent studies on Leap Motion sensor-based PD bradykinesia assessment

Depressed Sympathetic and Parasympathetic Cardiac Activity

Many PD patients present cardiac sympathetic denervation, particularly those with muscular rigidity and bradykinesia [109]. 20% of PD patients also suffer parasympathetic dysfunction that evolves into orthostatic hypotension [282, 325]. These dysfunctions are separate consequences of PD [119]. In theory, both could be monitored with heart-rate variability parameters such as the standard deviation of N-N intervals [57, 118, 147, 322]. Heart-rate variability alterations are a known risk factor for cardiovascular mortality [327]. These data could be acquired with photoplethysmography (PPG) [281].

PPG can detect heartbeats by analyzing changes in skin color. A smartphone can capture PPG signals by using the LED flash as a source of light and the camera as photoreceptor, when the user places their finger over the camera lens. The possibility of using smartphones for PPG has been previously discussed [87, 115, 116, 140]. This procedure can also be used to monitor blood pressure [39] and oxygen saturation [33]. If one were to extract frames from videos captured with the smartphone camera, for a given resolution, three values per pixel are captured (red, green and blue). Typically, PPG uses the green channel [198] since hemoglobin reflects most light in this wavelength. However, other channels should also be considered [326], since the green channel becomes useless if ambient light is low [176].

Smartphone cameras have been proven to accurately measure heart-rate at 30 Hz [250]. However, theoretically, a sampling rate of 200 Hz is required for heart-rate variability [331]. The possibility of using cubic spline interpolation, bandpass filtering [6] and signal derivatives has been discussed [66]. In this context, we found a limited number of studies comparing smartphone-based PPG with the gold standard, electrocardiography (ECG).

Blokhovsky et al. [25] conducted a comparison between ECG and PPG in 22 participants, using both 20 and 30 Hz smartphone cameras. They found correlations between 0.72 and 1, citing low framerates as the main issue. Peng et al. [244] compared sixteen heart-rate variability features between ECG and PPG in 30 users, obtaining correlations between 0.7 and 1, stating motion artifacts as the main confounder. Both authors mentioned manually editing signals in case heartbeats were skipped. In this book, we present a novel PPG algorithm that can accurately detect heartbeats and thus measure heart-rate and heart-rate variability. We also compare the accuracy of our algorithm with ECG. This algorithm is presented in *Chapter 7*, Section *Heart-rate Estimation Algorithm*.

Blink-rate

An additional dyskinesia factor in PD is its effect on eye blink-rate. This symptom has great interindividual variability and its mechanism is currently unknown. Several studies have reported lower blink-rates when comparing PD patients with healthy controls [22, 150, 309]. In addition, ON phases temporarily double the blink-rate in PD patients [163, 309]. This would suggest that it is possible to distinguish PD patients and healthy controls as well as ON and OFF periods of a PD patient based on the blink-rate. In [80], authors suggest a value of 20 blinks per minute or lower as a possible indicator of PD. Algorithms for blink detection to detect eye fatigue [58], or driver drowsiness [52] may also be used to monitor PD patients. To date, the best approach to detect eye blinks is to use the eye aspect ratio algorithm [290], combined with a support vector machine [186, 290]. In *Chapter 7*, Section *Blink-rate Estimation Algorithm*, we present a blink-rate detection algorithm based on the eye aspect ratio.

3.2. Exergame-based Interventions in Parkinson's Disease

In their 2014 systematic review, Barry et al. [18] analyzed the state of the art of exergame-based interventions in PD. They found a total of seven studies, one of which fulfilled the criteria for definition as a clinical trial. Authors mostly criticized methodological designs, and found that most studies were limited to analyzing feasibility and safety, and not potential therapeutic effects. However, they noted that, in the single clinical study identified, the exergame performed as well as traditional rehabilitation. We conducted a systematic review to expand on these findings. We searched for clinical and pilot trials published from 2014 onwards, with criteria based on Barry et al. [92]. This review was conducted in accordance with the PRISMA guidelines [221]. We qualified a study as a clinical trial if it fulfilled the CONSORT guidelines [280]. The databases of Pubmed, Scopus, Science Direct, IEEE and Cochrane were consulted by searching for studies published from January 1, 2014 to November 17, 2018 (the date of the last search). We used the final search string: *"Exergam* OR active video gaming OR Microsoft Kinect OR Kinect OR Nintendo Wii OR Wii OR Sony EyeToy OR IREX OR Dance Dance Revolution AND Parkinson*."* An asterisk represents all words that contain the character, regardless of termination.

This search yielded 526 matches at the last query, of which 353 were duplicates. We also excluded articles if (1) the target group was not exclusively PD (77 exclusions) or (2) the therapy employed was not exergame-based (32 exclusions). This resulted in 65 articles which were then classified into randomized clinical trials (9), pilot studies (11), non-evaluated concepts (30), and metastudies (15). We focused our study on clinical trials and pilot trials. After conducting this review and while implementing our approach, we included five additional publications concerning our topic. The complete results of this review are provided in *Appendix C*. We summarize these results as follows.

Researchers prefer the Microsoft Kinect to the Wii Balance Board, and we believe this is due to the versatility of the Kinect sensor. However, the Wii Balance Board presents positive results more consistently. Home-scenario implementations have been discussed [5, 289]. No studies showed worse outcomes in the exergaming group compared to the control group. We observed positive cognitive outcomes in some cases. Authors state that for cognitive training to be effective, it has to be a series of carefully planned tasks [247]. A summary of the results of our meta-analysis on clinical trials is provided in *Table 5*. From this meta-analysis, and based on standard statistical criteria ($p<0.05$ for statistical significance and $g>0.8$ for a large effect size) we draw the following conclusions. The following studies show measurable improvements in the intervention group: Liao et al. [194], Ribas et al. [268], Ferraz et al. [76], and Tollar et al. [316]. Unfortunately, the clinical outcomes of Ferraz et al. did not allow us to compare them in *Table 5*. The following studies show an improvement in the intervention group that is significantly higher than the control group: Liao et al. [194], Ribas et al. [268], and Tollar et al. [316]. In *Appendix C*, a complete table of studies is provided in *Table 43* and *Table 44*, and their effect sizes and statistical significance is presented in *Table 45* and *Table 46*.

Outcome: Timed Up-and-go Test (s) (lower is better)	N per group	Control method	Intervention method	Control Hedges's g (p), after-before	Intervention Hedges's g (p), after-before
Liao et al. [194]	12	Regular exercise	Wii Balance Board, commercial game	0.2034 (0.5954)	-0.8230 (0.0402)
Shih et al. [283]	11	Balance training	Kinect, custom game	-0.3371 (0.3990)	-0.1952 (0.6231)
Song et al. [289]	30	Usual healthcare	Dance mat, commercial game	-0.2443 (0.3479)	0.0663 (0.7983)
Outcome: Berg Balance Scale (adimensional) (higher is better)					
Pompeu et al. [252]	16	Balance training	Wii Balance Board, commercial game	0.2800 (0.4080)	0.4303 (0.2071)
Shih et al. [283]	11	Balance training	Kinect, custom game	0.4940 (0.2211)	0.6550 (0.1096)
Ribas et al. [268]	10	Regular exercise	Wii Balance Board, custom game	-0.0658 (0.8732)	0.6800 (0.1115)
Tollar et al. [316]	24/25 (control/intervention)	Usual healthcare	Kinect, commercial game	-0.2420 (0.3885)	2.1277 (<0.0001)

Table 5: Summarized meta-analysis of clinical trials concerning exergame-based PD interventions

Pilot trials also provided interesting results. All studies reported improvements in clinical outcomes. The possibility of remote monitoring has also been discussed [7]. This study also provides a direct comparison between the Wii Balance Board and Kinect sensors. However, results of this study do not allow us to draw definite conclusions, since effect sizes are similar. A summary of the most relevant results of our meta-analysis on pilot trials is provided in *Table 6*. Although they do not allow for a direct comparison of results, both Goncalves et al. [110] and Negrini et al. [231] show statistically significant improvements. In *Appendix C*, a complete set of studies is provided in *Table 47* and *Table 48*,and their effect sizes and statistical significance is available in *Table 49*.

We found a number of limitations in the methodologies of these articles. First, many studies did not use standard clinical outcomes, which meant we could not include them in our meta-analysis. Second, mild cognitive impairment was mentioned as an exclusion criterion in all studies. Thus, the feasibility of this approach in this cohort is unknown. The importance of adapting the games to the user's skills was also frequently mentioned, but not always implemented. In summary, out of 19 studies including an evaluation, 17 indicate improvements in PD patients when playing exergames. In the case of clinical trials, seven out of nine report better results in the exergaming group compared to the control group. In the remaining two studies, both groups had equal results. Exergames also seem to have a positive impact on cognition. The safety and feasibility of game-based PD rehabilitation were confirmed, and the first insight into its superiority to traditional rehabilitation was provided. However, these results are mostly statistically non-significant, due to low sample sizes. Effect sizes do suggest that larger studies would provide more substantial evidence.

Outcome: Timed Up-and-go Test (s) (lower is better)	N	Intervention method	Hedges's g (p), after-before
Summa et al. [303]	7	Kinect, custom game	0.0638 (0.8927)
Alves et al. [7]	9	Wii Balance Board, commercial game	-0.3235 (0.4558)
Alves et al. [7]	9	Kinect, commercial game	-0.3788 (0.3841)
Outcome: 10-Meter Walk Test (s) (lower is better)			
Palacios et al. [240]	7	Kinect, custom game	-0.3139 (0.5109)
Summa et al. [303]	7	Kinect, custom game	0 (1)
Alves et al. [7]	9	Wii Balance Board, commercial game	-0.0962 (0.8230)
Alves et al. [7]	9	Kinect, commercial game	-0.0691 (0.8724)

Table 6: Summarized meta-analysis of pilot trials concerning exergame-based PD interventions

We complemented this systematic review with studies using the Leap Motion sensor [72, 237, 238, 276]. In [238], a battery of Leap-Motion based exergames for PD rehabilitation was designed, where patients perform hand movements such as grabbing or pinching. Authors state the importance of scenario adaptability, for example, the number of repetitions, or thresholds to determine when a pinching or grabbing movement is performed. A pilot trial with five PD patients showed improvements in game performance: patients took less time to complete the same exercise after a few sessions. This improvement translated into hand grip strength, hand dexterity and eye-hand coordination. A second, trial with 23 participants produced similar results [72]. Authors are exploring the possibility of including VR, also with promising results [237, 276].

We identified a number of limitations in this study. First, it is necessary to extend exergame-based interventions to other PD areas, such as hand dexterity. Other authors discuss this as well [82]. Second, the potential role of exergames as a monitoring system should be explored. Our work in this regard further underlines the importance of task specificity and scenario adaptability.

3.3. Other Game-based Interventions

Brain-Computer Interfaces

The use of BCIs in PD has been discussed as a potential method to monitor the effectivity of deep brain stimulation [196]. It could also be potentially employed for cognitive training [184], cognitive assessment [32], as well as general rehabilitation procedures [46]. The possibility of implementing a serious game controlled by a brain computer interface has also been explored [193]. Unfortunately, classification accuracy when estimating, for example, directional intention, is quite low [78] except when aiming to classify binary choices [178]. In this book, we explore the possibility of using an electroencephalographic device to control a serious game to train concentration. This is discussed in *Chapter 8*, section *Brain-Computer Interfaces*.

Virtual Reality

Recent studies have explored the possibility of extending exergame-based interventions in PD to VR [317]. This has the same positive effects as traditional exergames [43, 205]. However, VR significantly increases player immersion [35, 36]. Hereby, motion sickness in VR, also known as cybersickness, is a very significant problem. Most VR users experience cybersickness [47, 162, 265, 266, 271, 294] after 10 minutes [179]. Its cause is still disputed. Literature defines it as a sensory conflict between vision and proprioception, mediated by the perception of self-motion, also known as vection [125, 181, 286]. However, the exact relation between cybersickness and vection is not known [153, 157, 264]. A number of secondary factors are also discussed in the literature. Adaptability [222, 223, 293], the nature of VR movements [199, 214, 224, 288, 300], controllability [156, 273, 295], technical factors such as latency, jitter, and field of view [37, 67, 129, 155, 181, 299] contribute to cybersickness. User adaptation seems to be the best strategy at the moment [138].

A possibility to detect cybersickness is to study its physiological effects. Cybersickness has been reported to increases cortisol levels [152], cause tachycardia [131, 133], increase sweating [138], and change heart-rate variability [269]. However, individual responses in autonomic regulation make it difficult to predict cybersickness based exclusively on said physical responses [165]. Based on these data, the literature suggests that galvanic skin response (sweating) may be the best approach [55, 95, 100, 101, 229]. However, a potential increase in accuracy when considering additional data sources (such as head movements) remains to be performed. This situation sets a scenario similar to the one discussed in this book. It could be possible to use game data, data from the VR device and physiological data to detect cybersickness as a symptom. We discuss this possibility in *Chapter 8*, section *Virtual Reality*.

4. Model for an Exergame-based Clinical Decision Support System

To address the research gap presented in *Chapter 1,* and based on our findings in *Chapter 3,* we now describe the components of an exergame-based clinical decision support system model designed to monitor a symptom of a chronic disease. In this chapter, we also describe the materials and methods required to realize it. This model uses standard clinical assessments as ground truth to validate the accuracy of its predictions, and should extract clinically meaningful data from the players using sensors and game data. To the player, this model is presented as an exergame, where data acquisition occurs in the background of the game. We conceive such a model as a technical data acquisition module that extracts data from the exergame, the sensors used to operate it, and the players themselves. This produces three data streams: game data, interaction data, and biosignals. These data streams are processed in different manners into feature vectors. These feature vectors, combined with standard clinical assessments extracted from health records (or measured during the evaluation), produce a single feature vector per patient. A clinical decision support system, trained on the standard clinical assessment, then produces clinically meaningful data. Specific implementations, as proofs of concept of the model, for the scenarios of balance and tremor are described in *Chapter 5* and *Chapter 6,* and potential biosignal acquisition systems are described in *Chapter 7.* We also discuss the materials and methods we used in these implementations. Finally, we describe the ethical risks and considerations we identified and addressed when conducting our research.

4.1. Model Design

The design of our model can be summarized as follows. A patient plays an exergame using a sensor (or sensors) that is also used to monitor a target symptom (or symptoms) of PD: in the specific cases of this book, hand tremors and balance. The exergame contains a certain physical and cognitive challenge. The model collects data from three separate sources: the exergame, the sensors used to control the game, and facultatively, the players themselves. We define these data sources as game data, interaction data, and biosignals. From these data, a series of features are extracted. The combination of these features produces a feature vector per patient as a result.

This feature vector is processed by a series of classifiers into estimations that can be used to assess the severity of the symptom in question. In this book, we refer to such estimations as clinically meaningful data. These data provide relevant, objective clinical information in absolute terms (e.g., is the patient at an increased risk of falling?) or in relative terms (e.g., is the current physical rehabilitation improving balance?). A caregiver can use these data as a source of information in addition to their clinical standards, for example UPDRS. This provides them with more objective data when making clinical decisions, such as adapting the current medication or rehabilitation plan.

To evaluate and train our clinical decision support system, we take the clinical standards employed in medical practice into account. We use the 30 Second Sit-To-Stand test [270] to assess balance and the risk of falling, and UPDRS to assess hand tremor and bradykinesia. The goal of the methods presented in this book is not to replace these standards, but to complement them by providing an additional objective data source that could be provided remotely. The evaluations included in this book use these standards as ground truth to justify the validity of the presented systems.

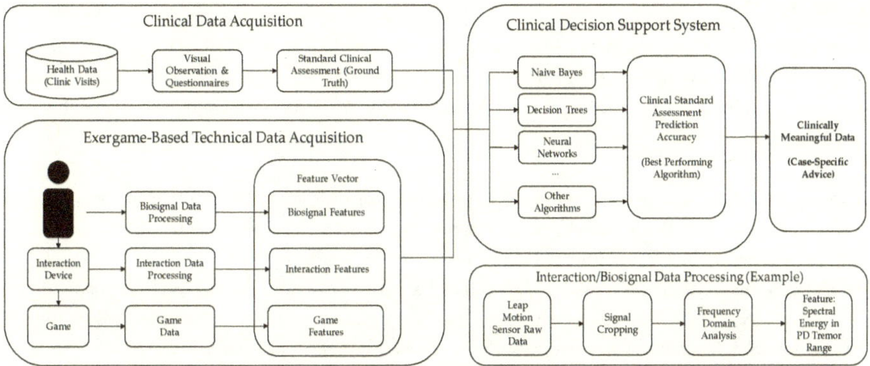

Figure 4: Model diagram of an exergame-based clinical decision support system

As presented in *Figure 4*, the model consists of a data acquisition module, comprised of the game, interaction device, and the players themselves. This module produces the three data streams. These streams are processed separately into features using different techniques. These features are then combined, together with the standard clinical assessment, into the feature vector. This feature vector is processed in a clinical decision support system, producing a certain classification result, producing the clinically meaningful data. The following sections describe data processing, classification, and the specific materials and methods we employed in this book. Implementations of this concept are presented in *Chapter 5* and *Chapter 6*.

4.2. Data Processing and Classification

Data processing refers to all procedures employed towards converting a data source, for example raw data from an accelerometer, into a feature vector. There is a number of differences in the processing of different data sources. Game data requires no filtering and can generally be used directly as features. Both interaction data and biosignals usually require filtering and processing, which is defined on a case-by-case basis. Biosignals are facultative to the application scenario.

Game Data

Game Data refers to all data collected directly from the exergame. These consist of a series of variables that refer to the player's performance. Examples of game data are the time needed to finish a level or the maximum difficulty level achieved. These data are simple to extract and rarely require filtering or processing. Thus, they are usually included in the feature vector as-is.

Game features refer to how the players have performed in the game. This includes information on how much time they required to solve each level, how many actions they performed, and the nature of these actions. For example, when solving a puzzle, a comparison between the number of movements a player did and the minimum number of necessary movements provides relevant cognitive information. Features related to difficulty also contain information on the physical and cognitive skills of the player. For that purpose, data, such as the maximum level of difficulty achieved, or how performance changes with increasing difficulty, are relevant.

Interaction Data

Interaction data refers to features extracted from raw sensor data measuring the interactions of the player with the exergame in the form of physical movements. These physical movements operate the exergame. Examples of interaction data are hand movements or physical steps used to navigate a map or solve a puzzle.

These type of data require different forms of processing prior to feature extraction, such as filtering or frequency domain analysis, which are established on a case-by-case basis. In this book, we use finite impulse response bandpass filters. For example, when analyzing hand movements, the 3-15 Hz frequency range contains relevant information on hand tremors [219]. This can be combined with other techniques, such as moving average filters, or peak detection algorithms. Once filtered, both time- and frequency-domain analysis is performed. Time-domain analysis produces features, such as means, standard deviations, amplitudes, speeds, and accelerations. Conversely, frequency-domain analysis provides information on the spectral components of the signal in different frequency ranges.

Biosignals

Biosignals refer to any electrical (e.g., ECG) or non-electrical (e.g., PPG) signal measured from the player's body. These signals can be acquired with or without physical contact [228]. Their processing, and the features to be extracted from them, are established on a case-by-case basis. For example, in ECG, one may use a peak detection algorithm to time heartbeats, and calculate the heart-rate. This heart-rate can then be used to estimate exertion [201]. Alternatively, more sophisticated features, such as negative T-wave [200] detection, can be used to diagnose cardiopathies [332]. The devices employed to collect biosignals also vary greatly. For example, it is possible to use a relatively cheap smartphone or an expensive biosignal amplifier to measure PPG signals [90]. The development of more cost-efficient methods to acquire biosignals and clinically meaningful data represents a research field in itself [15].

Within our concept, it is possible to include additional biosignals that could be collected while exergaming to monitor additional PD symptoms. In *Chapter 7, Heart-rate Estimation Algorithm* and *Blink-rate Estimation Algorithm*, we present two novel biosignal acquisition methods that are of clinical relevance in PD. In both cases, we employ peak- and zero-crossing detection algorithms, and produce both time- and frequency-domain features, such as heart-rate variability features.

Classification

The feature vectors produced by the data processing methods can then be classified to estimate a clinical outcome. For example, the goal of the system presented in *Chapter 5* is to predict whether the player is at an increased risk of falling. A clinical standard to assess this possibility is the 30-Second-Sit-to-Stand Test. Thus, the goal when evaluating this system is to predict the outcome of said test based on game data, interaction data, and biosignals. For this purpose, numerous classification techniques and classifier algorithms can be employed. In most cases, once a classification problem is defined (e.g., detect outliers, linear regression, logistic regression) several algorithms are tested (e.g., Naïve Bayes, J48, Neural Networks [204]). We complete this analysis with an evaluation of statistical significance and effect sizes.

4.3. Implementation Materials and Methods

In this section, we describe the nonspecific materials and methods used in this book. Specific hardware devices are described in *Chapter 5, Chapter 6,* and *Chapter 7*. Most of the hardware used in this book is based on commercial off-the-shelf devices. We intended for our implemented systems to be cost-effective. We also decided to design systems in which the patient does not have to wear any equipment on themselves, thus avoiding wearables, whenever possible. The exception to this rule was biosignal acquisition. We acquired biosignals using smartphones and the g.USBAmp biosignal amplifier developed by g.Tec [85]. This particular device was chosen due to its accuracy and array of available measurement devices, including active electrodes. Active electrodes were important to deliver signals free of movement artifacts and other noise sources such as sweating.

All prototypically implemented exergames were initially developed using Kha [170], a Haxe-based open source multimedia framework created by Robert Konrad. The main advantage of Kha over other development tools is its cross-platform capability. This allowed us to rapidly publish the games in several platforms, such as web browsers, Windows and Unity [321].

All data processing, filtering, and feature extraction procedures were performed in Matlab [210]. We chose Matlab because of our previous experience with it and its toolbox support, particularly the graphical programming environment Simulink. It also offers toolboxes to address most of the technical tasks in this book, such as finite impulse response filters and frequency domain analysis. We imported our data sources into Matlab using different methods. If data were not received in real-time, we stored it in a format that is readable in Matlab, for example XML, CSV or JSON.

Classification tasks were performed in Weka [204]. Although Matlab includes a machine learning toolbox, we preferred Weka because it provides a wider array of options. For each classification problem, we use all of the algorithms provided by Weka that are suitable for the problem in question. We provide summarized versions of these results concerning the best performing algorithms. In general, our classification problems refer to binary supervised learning problems. In binary classification situations, we always define the intervention group (e.g., PD patients) as the positive group. In this circumstance, considering we are implementing a medical system, our priority is to ensure that no members of the intervention group are misclassified as healthy. Thus, our criterion to define the "best" algorithms is to prioritize a minimization of False Negatives (FN), while also considering the remaining factors. For each classifier, we present the following characteristics of the two best performing algorithms: Accuracy (% of correct classifications), confusion matrix including True Positives (TP), FN, True Negatives (TN) and False Positives (FP), TP rate (recall), FP rate, precision, F-measure, Matthews Correlation Coefficient (MCC), area under the Receiver Operating Characteristic curve (ROC area), and Precision/Recall (PRC) area. We also include the accuracy (% of correct classifications) results of all the employed algorithms. Unless otherwise specified, we use 10-fold cross validation. A complete list of algorithm hyperparameters is provided in *Appendix D, Table 50,* and a description of the classifier characteristics is included in *Table 51*.

In addition to classification results, we provide data on statistical significance and effect sizes. We use Shapiro-Wilk to test for normality [263]. If the sample in question follows a normal distribution, we use a Welch t-test to evaluate statistical significance. If not, we use Kolmogorov-Smirnov [27]. The effect size is a measure of the magnitude of the presented results. We chose Hedges's g [123] using low sample size bias correction as a measure of effect size. This parameter is very frequently used in literature and is specifically designed for varying sample sizes and groups with different standard deviations, in comparison to other measures such as Cohen's d [48] or Glass's delta [122]. These effect sizes are generally interpreted using Cohen's rule of thumb [48] as "small" (0.2), "medium" (0.5) and "large" (0.8), although the terms depend on the circumstances of the study. In this book, effect sizes are always calculated as $after - before$ and $intervention - control$. This means a positive effect size reveals an increase in the measured factor after the procedure or in the intervention group in comparison with the control group. In order to calculate the number of participants required for studies with two groups, we used the sample size calculation formula presented in [143]. We employ the median standard deviation and consider 80% power and an effect size of 0.65 with a significance level of 0.05. A complete list of these calculations is provided in *Table 52*.

4.4. Ethical Considerations

The evaluation of this book includes methods that required the collection of personal and physiological data. Specifically, we identified the following potential ethical issues in this book:

- Ethical issues related to the acquisition of biometric data from PD patients and healthy controls regarding their physiological status: hand tremors, gait, and biosignals.
- Ethical issues related to the acquisition of personal information via questionnaires and medical reports: age, sex, details of neurodegenerative or otherwise chronic diseases, medication plans.
- Ethical issues related to ensuring the privacy and anonymity of the aforementioned data

We carefully considered these ethical issues, and before commencing evaluation procedures we obtained approval of the ethics committee of the Technical University of Darmstadt. In addition, since part of the evaluation took place in the State of Baden-Wüttemberg, we also sought approval of the ethics committee of the University Medical Centre Mannheim. The complete list of votes of ethical committees for evaluations in this book is included in *Appendix D, Table 53*.

In pursuance of the declaration of Helsinki addressing ethical principles for medical research involving human subjects [13], the studies presented in this book are limited to voluntary participants. Prior to participation, users were asked to read and sign an informed consent. This document described the procedure, data collected, how these data would be used, and our research goal in understandable language. All data collected in this book is pseudonymized through randomized user numbers assigned to non-identifiable data and cannot be backtracked to the participants. The informed consents for both evaluation scenarios are provided in *Appendix E* and *Appendix F* in German language. For each evaluation scenario, the cohort is adjusted to the study parameters, and the size of the cohort is based on candidates that fulfilled the specified inclusion and exclusion criteria. Due to the COVID-19 pandemic and stay-at-home regulations, visits to PD patients in clinics were strictly forbidden. This meant we had to adjust or delay many evaluation plans. For this reason, the cohort of *Chapter 5* was changed to nursing home residents. In *Chapter 6,* it was essential to perform the evaluation with PD patients. We present the results of a preliminary study for this scenario.

5. Design of an Exergame-based Clinical Decision Support System to Assess Balance

Based on our model for an exergame-based clinical decision support system described in *Chapter 4*, in this chapter we present and evaluate a proof of concept of this model to assess balance. First, two different hardware approaches to acquire data are presented. The first approach consists of an array of six Wii Balance Boards, called Extended Balance Board. Compared to the Wii Balance Board, this array allowed us to create a larger surface with which to evaluate balance both while standing and walking, and was published in [88]. The second approach includes two further biosignals: back muscle activity and upper trunk rotation while walking. We designed this more complex system to evaluate the possibility of using additional data sources. This system was published in [168]. We tested this system with a cohort of 40 participants with gait and balance affections, with the goal of identifying characteristic differences in muscular activity and upper trunk rotation. Since our preliminary results in this cohort did not indicate that we would obtain better results than using the center of mass only, we implemented our final design using the Extended Balance Board. After concluding our data acquisition design, we created a novel dual-tasking exergame entitled PDDanceCity. This exergame uses the Extended Balance Board as a control device to navigate a labyrinth and presents a motor and cognitive task to the player. PDDanceCity was published in [91]. We concluded our system design with an evaluation. This evaluation took place with 16 participants from an elderly nursing home in Darmstadt. The goal of this evaluation was to perform a binary prediction of the risk of falling, using the clinical outcome of the 30-Second-Sit-To-Stand Test [270] as ground truth. This test establishes whether the subject is likely to have an age-average fall risk (fit, over the threshold) or an increased risk (not fit, under the threshold). We use game data (data from PDDanceCity) and interaction data (data from the Extended Balance Board) to predict if the player is under or over this threshold. Our classification results indicate that the system can accurately indicate if a player is at an age- and sex-adjusted increased risk of falling. This evaluation is published in [20]. Further experimental details are available in *Appendix E*. We conclude this chapter with an acceptance test of PDDanceCity. Potential users found the game to be user-friendly and fun. They also found the difficulty levels to be well-adjusted to their skills.

5.1. Data Acquisition

In the section *Assessing Balance and Gait* of *Chapter 3*, we present two studies [215, 342] that indicate the Wii Balance Board could be used to discriminate patients with an increased risk of falling. In the section *Exergame-based Interventions in Parkinson's Disease*, we identified two clinical trials [194, 268] and two pilot trials [110, 231] showing a positive effect when using the Wii Balance Board in PD patients. We also identified two clinical trials [76, 316] and one pilot trial [253] using the Kinect sensor with a similar result. This may suggest that both are viable approaches for our design. However, the number of studies using the Kinect sensor were significantly higher (12 studies used the Kinect, and 5 used the Wii Balance Board, see *Table 42*). This meant that more studies using the Kinect sensor had resulted in non-significant results compared to the Wii Balance Board, indicating the Wii Balance Board may be a slightly better approach. For this reason, we decided to use the Wii Balance Board for our design.

As also discussed in the section *Assessing Balance and Gait*, PD affects balance both while standing and walking. The surface of the Wii Balance Board, which we measured to be 25.5-by-44 cm, does not provide a large enough surface to analyze several steps. For this reason, we decided to use an array of six Wii Balance Boards. We called this system Extended Balance Board.

In order to design the Extended Balance Board, we had to access the data of each Wii Balance Board. The Wii Balance Board consists of the following components: An electronic control unit, battery housing, power button, and four sensors, one in each corner (*Figure 5*). With the data from these four sensors, it is possible to determine the weight on the board and its distribution [314]. Thus, the Extended Balance Board would provide us with a surface of 76.5 by 88 cm, and 24 piezoelectric sensors distributed across this surface. We needed to acquire the data from all six Wii Balance Boards simultaneously and send them to a computer. For this purpose, we designed a controller board, called Acquisition Serializer Board. This board collects the data from each Wii Balance Board via Bluetooth and sends it, combined with information about which board the sensor belongs to, to a computer via serial port. This system was presented in [88].

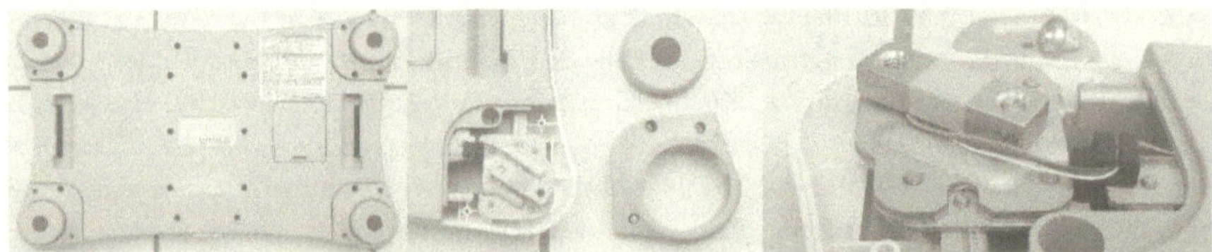

Figure 5: Wii Balance Board sensors

Each Wii Balance Board communicates through a duplex Bluetooth channel. The first channel transmits control commands (input) and the second channel provides sensor information (output). This means the Acquisition Serializer Board must simultaneously establish twelve Bluetooth communication channels: six boards, with two channels each. To make this possible, the board uses two Blue-1000 Bluetooth sticks [203] that permit a maximum of eight connections each. The controller board ensures continuous communication despite the inherent stability and latency issues, mainly by circumventing the radio channels using the Universal Asynchronous Receiver/Transmitter interfaces. The Wii Balance Board data are decoded using the WiiUse Library [177] according to the instructions provided in [340] by the Acquisition Serializer Board, with a frequency of approximately 20 Hz per board. These data include both sensor values (11 bytes) and calibration values (32 bytes). A description of the data format of the Wii Balance Board is provided in *Table 7*.

The exact weight detected by each sensor, in kg, is calculated by the Acquisition Serializer Board, based on the sensor and calibration values (*Table 7)* provided by the Wii Balance Board. The Wii Balance Board provides the values for three reference measured weights: 0 kg, 17 kg and 34 kg (the latter being the maximum weight the sensor can measure). The weight calculation works by interpolating the sensor data and the calibration values. For example, if the actual sensor value is 4800 and the calibration values are [2000,5000,8000], representing $[0kg, 17kg, 34kg]$, then the actual measured sensor weight would be:

$$Sensor\ weight\ (kg) = 17 \cdot \frac{4800 - 2000}{5000 - 2000} = 15.87\ kg$$

Sensor data - Byte	Content	Calibration data – Byte	Content
0	Top right <15:8>	0x20	Unknown, always 0x01
1	Top right <7:0>	0x21	Reference battery level (always 0x69)
2	Bottom right <15:8>	0x22, 0x23	0
3	Bottom right <7:0>	0x24	Top right 0kg value <15:8>
4	Top left <15:8>	0x25	Top right 0 kg value <7:0>
5	Top left <7:0>	0x26, 0x27	Bottom right 0kg value
6	Bottom left <15:8>	0x28, 0x29	Top left 0kg value
7	Bottom left <7:0>	0x2A, 0x2B	Bottom left 0kg value
8	Temperature	0x2C-0x33	17 kg values
9	0	0x34-0x3B	34 kg values
10	Battery level	0x3C-0x3F	CRC32 checksum

Table 7: Wii Balance Board sensor and calibration data composition [340]

The PC then receives the processed data. These data include the sensor values and a unique board identifier, linked to the MAC Address of each Wii Balance Board. This is done to identify the board sending data, since each one has a specific position in the Extended Balance Board (*Table 8*). The total weight is calculated as the sum of the sensor weights.

Data type	Description	Example
Int	MAC	58bda3a9cd6f
Int	Board ID	3
Float (4)	Sensor weights (top left, top right, bottom left, bottom right)	30.022, 26.871, 16.940, 16.052
Int (4)	Sensor values (top left, top right, bottom left, bottom right)	10265, 5522, 4800, 9157
Float	Total weight (kg)	89.887

Table 8: Sample of a data packet received from the Acquisition Serializer Board [88]

This procedure allowed us to receive real-time data on how a player is standing on the board, and how they shift their weight when standing and when taking a step. We still needed to transform these data into parameters that allowed us to control an exergame. We decided to do this by calculating a bidimensional projection (x, y) of the Center of Mass ($\boldsymbol{com}$) based on sensor positions and values. This is done by multiplying the sensor values by its bidimensional coordinates, as follows:

Let $\mathbf{S} \in \mathbb{R}^{6\times4}$ be the matrix of sensor values (3×2 Wii Balance Boards, with four sensors each). Let $\mathbf{S}(t)$ be the matrix of sensor values at the discrete sampling time t, and thus $s_{\mathrm{i,j}}(t)$ the value of sensor $s_{\mathrm{i,j}}$ at this discrete sampling time t. Let $\mathbf{C} \in \mathbb{R}^{6\times4\times2}$ be the coordinate matrix, containing two-dimensional (x, y) vectors assigning a coordinate value to each sensor position. This position is based on its placement on the board, measured in relative terms to the actual frame dimensions (i.e. $\boldsymbol{c}_{1,1} = (-1,1)$

as described in *Figure 6*). Finally, let $w(t)$ be the latest weight value, calculated by the Acquisition Serializer Board as the sum of all board weights as described in *Table 8*. The instantaneous center of mass vector at the discrete sampling time t, $\boldsymbol{com}(t)$ can be calculated as:

$$\boldsymbol{com}(t) = (com_x(t), com_y(t)) = \frac{1}{w(t)} \sum_{i=1}^{6} \sum_{j=1}^{4} (s_{i,j}(t)\boldsymbol{c}_{i,j})$$

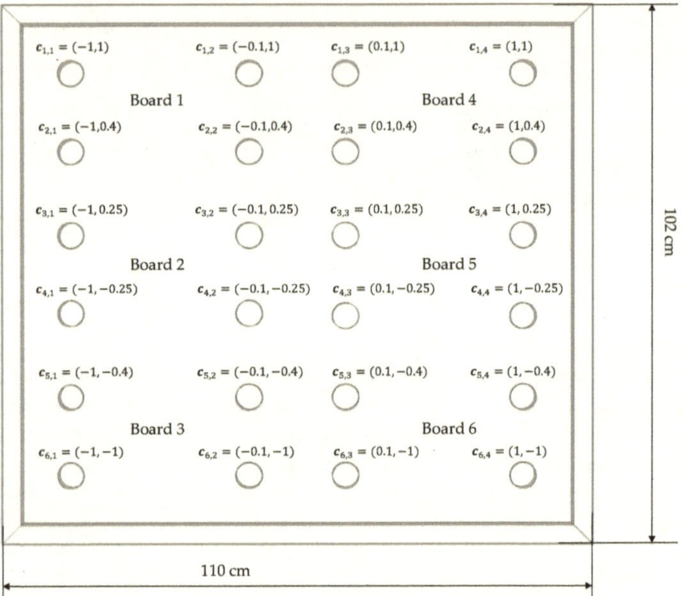

Figure 6: Extended Balance Board distribution and coordinate matrix **C**, presented in [20, 88]. Each hole fits one of the feet of the respective Wii Balance Board

A sample of the $\boldsymbol{com}$ when taking a step is presented in *Figure 7*. The $\boldsymbol{com}$ is normalized using the player's weight, and can be used to estimate intention. Its values are in the range $com_x, com_y \in [-1,1]$. In this range, we use the value 0.5 as a threshold for directional intention. Given the values of **C**, this limit worked well as a threshold for directional intention. More specifically, a value of 0.5 or greater in a direction, combined with a value of 0.1 or lower in the other coordinate indicates a directional intention. For instance, $\boldsymbol{com}(t) = (0.1, 0.8)$ indicates an intention to move upwards, while $\boldsymbol{com}(t) = (0.5, 0.8)$ is ignored. This parameter can be also used as a measure of balance [275]. It can also be calibrated on an individual basis, depending on the user's mobility. Every time that the Acquisition Serializer Board sends an update from a Wii Balance Board (that is, every instant t), the $\boldsymbol{com}$ is calculated again, which means it has a refresh rate of approximately 120 Hz.

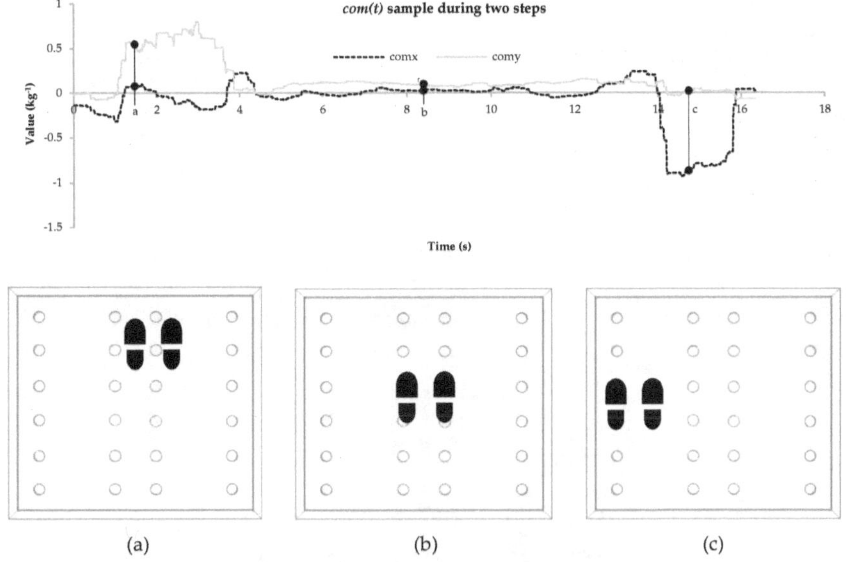

Figure 7: Sample of ***com*** (top) and feet position (bottom) when taking a forward step (point "a"), standing in the middle ("b") and taking a leftwards step ("c")

Besides the ***com***, we extract a second parameter from the board data, as a measure of the balance and lower extremity fitness of the player. This parameter is defined as the Instability Factor $if(t)$, and calculated as the root mean square of the first order difference of ***com***, as follows: let $\boldsymbol{com}(t)$ be defined as above, and $\boldsymbol{com}(t-1)$ be the value at the discrete sampling time $t-1$, so that $t > t-1$ and there is no sampling point in between, $\nexists\, t': t > t' > t-1$., then $if(t)$ at sampling point t can be calculated as:

$$if(t) = \sqrt{\frac{1}{2}(com_x(t) - com_x(t-1))^2 + \frac{1}{2}\,(com_y(t) - com_y(t-1))^2}$$

The if is in the range $if(t) \in [0,2]$. If the player does not move, this means $if(t) = 0$. If the player suddenly shifts their weight greatly, more so if they do so diagonally, the value of $if(t)$ increases up to a maximum of 2, which is only achievable if the player is at a corner and jumps to the opposite one. In reasonable terms, values of up to one can be expected for either a person with a great balance who takes very large steps, or a person that is losing balance. The $if(t)$ value can be compared with a threshold value (e.g., 0.5, or 1) and, if its value overcomes the said threshold, a possible loss of balance will be marked in the data. In general terms, slow and balanced movements would not trigger this threshold. Conversely, tripping will easily lead to exceeding this threshold for several frames in most cases. As is the case with intention estimation based on ***com*** values, it is also possible to calibrate the threshold on an individual basis. The specific processing diagram, as a part of the approach described in *Figure 4*, is presented in *Figure 8*. The final version of the Extended Balance Board is depicted in *Figure 9*.

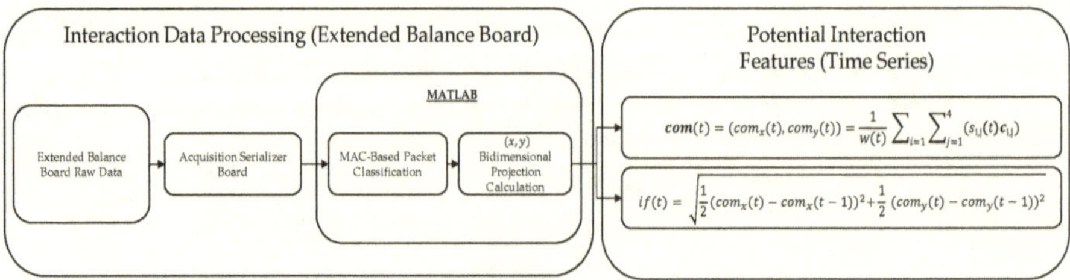

Figure 8: Extended Balance Board interaction data processing diagram

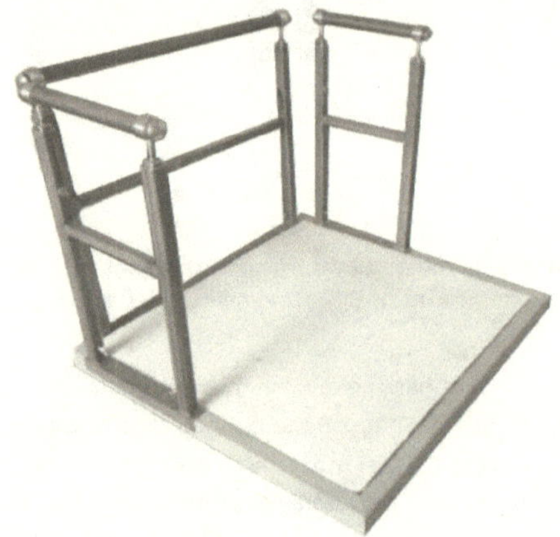

Figure 9: Extended Balance Board, presented in [20, 88]

Alternative Balance Assessment System

We also developed a second approach of a clinical decision support system to assess balance based on a combination of a laboratory pressure plate, triaxial accelerometers and electromyography. The goal of this alternative system, as an alternative to the Extended Balance Board, was to test its feasibility to identify more sophisticated biomarkers related to gait and balance affections. In a similar fashion, the system was conceived to identify these differences in signals acquired while participants with affected balance and gait stood on the pressure plate and walked over it.

This system comprises a Kistler 9287C8 force plate [166], two smartphones to measure relative rotation and forward acceleration, bipolar surface electromyography of the back muscles, and a piezoelectric step sensor. Both the electromyographic and the step signal were collected using the g.Tec USBAmp biosignal amplifier when standing, and its portable version, the Mobilab Bluetooth biosignal amplifier [85] when walking.

The Kistler Force Plate was connected to its own biosignal amplifier, and data was sent to the computer separately. We developed an application in Microsoft Visual Studio [218], based on code provided by Kistler in their proprietary library BioWare Dataserver [167]. This application collects the data from the Kistler biosignal amplifier. Its raw data consists of the three-dimensional forces $(F_x(t_{fp}), F_y(t_{fp}), F_z(t_{fp}))$ measured by the plate, for each discrete sampling time of the force plate t_{fp}, sampled at 1024 Hz. These data were sent to Matlab. From these forces, and including the user's weight w, we calculated the root mean square of the center of mass (rms_{COM}). We also calculated the vertical forces at the point where the participant's heel touched the floor ($t_{fp} = heelstrike$) and was lifted from the floor ($t_{fp} = heeloff$). The identification of these points is performed with the piezoelectric sensor and described below. When analyzing the data in Matlab, we interpolated the sampling times of the force plate with those of the electromyographic data using cubic spline interpolation. A sample of this signal while walking is presented in *Figure 10*. The two peaks indicate $HSMAX$ and $HOMAX$.

$$rms_{COM}(t_{fp}) = \frac{1}{w}\sqrt{\frac{1}{3}\left(F_x(t_{fp})^2 + F_y(t_{fp})^2 + F_z(t_{fp})^2\right)} \text{ after cubic spline interpolation } rms_{COM}(t)$$

$$HSMAX = \frac{F_z}{w}(t_{fp} = heelstrike),\ HOMAX = \frac{F_z}{w}(t_{fp} = heeloff), \text{ after cubic spline interpolation using } t$$

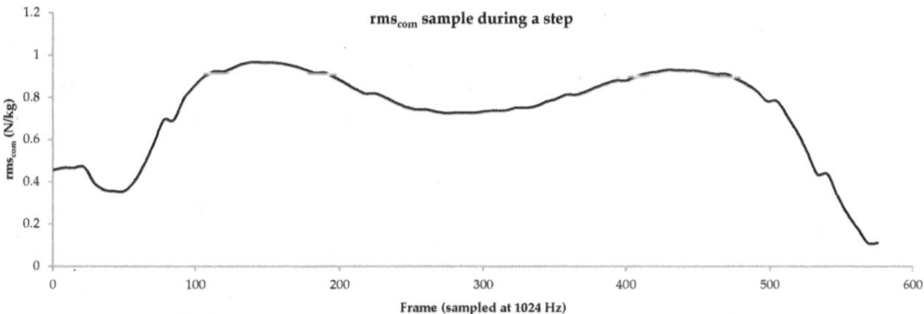

Figure 10: Sample of rms_{COM} during a step

The smartphone data was acquired using an application developed by us in Android Studio [112]. The application gathers the orientation and accelerometer sensor data as described in [113] at a sampling frequency of 100 Hz. It then sends it to the computer. We only used this procedure to ensure the smartphone was gathering data correctly, as we saved the sensor data locally. For our analysis, we used these locally stored data. To measure rotation, we collected all values of the difference of the smartphone above the hip, sampled at the time points of the smartphone t_s, $\vartheta_1(t_s)$ minus the one below $\vartheta_2(t_s)$. This is the angular position of the upper trunk relatively to the lower trunk. The position of the smartphones is depicted in *Figure 11*. To measure forward acceleration, we use the accelerometer z axis. When standing, only the rotation data are used, since no forward advance is expected. When walking, only the values between $heelstrike$ and $heeloff$, from both rotation and forward acceleration, were considered. When analyzing the data in Matlab, we interpolated the sampling times of the smartphones with those of the electromyographic data using cubic spline interpolation. Samples for both signals are presented in *Figure 12*.

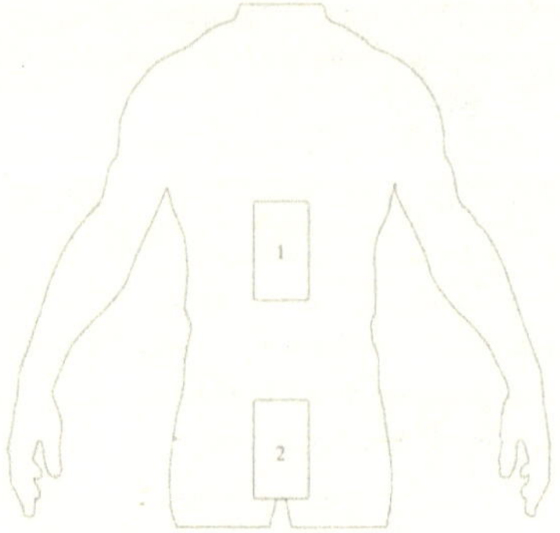

Figure 11: Smartphone placement to measure trunk rotation and acceleration. Courtesy of [195]

$$\vartheta(t_s) = |\vartheta_1(t_s) - \vartheta_2(t_s)|, \text{ after cubic spline interpolation } \vartheta(t)$$
$$a(t_s) = \frac{1}{2}|a_1(t_s) + a_2(t_s)|, \text{ after cubic spline interpolation } a(t)$$

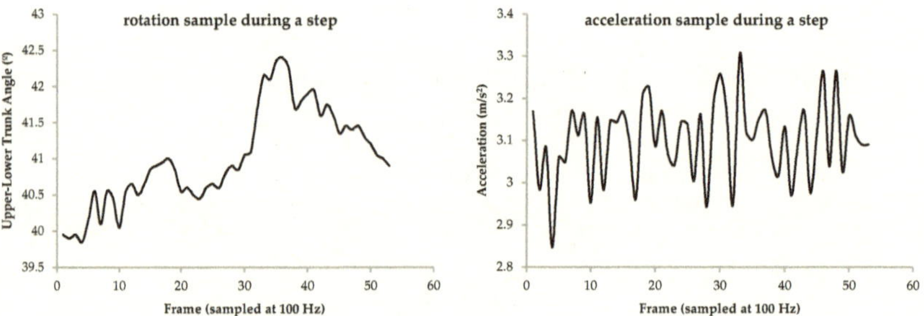

Figure 12: Rotation and acceleration sample during a step

The electromyographic signal was acquired using solid gel electrodes, placed bilaterally with an interelectrode distance of 23mm placed on the left and right side, lateral to the first lumbar processus spinosus. The placement of electrodes is depicted in *Figure 13*. Electromyographic data were acquired using the USBAmp biosignal amplifier, at a frequency of 1024 Hz, or the mobile version, the Mobilab Bluetooth biosignal amplifier, sampled at 256 Hz. A 50 Hz notch filter was employed, followed by a 17 to 500 Hz bandpass filter (replaced by a 17 Hz highpass filter in case the Mobilab was used). We employed a Simulink module developed by g.Tec to collect data in Matlab directly. In the standing scenario, the whole sample was considered. When analyzing gait, we only considered the data between $heelstrike$ and $heeloff$. Since both erector spinae muscles were measured, we referred to the right side as $emg_R(t)$ and the left side as $emg_L(t)$. In addition, a normalization procedure was included. Data was divided by the maximum value of erector spinae activity when lying in prone position, with the knees flexed backwards 90 degrees, and lifting the legs five cm over the surface, as described in [53, 159]. This value is defined as EMG_{Max} for each side. We used the sampling points of the electromyographic data as the basis for all data analysis. A sample of this signal is presented in *Figure 14*.

$$emg(t) = (\frac{emg_R(t)}{EMG_{R_{Max}}}, \frac{emg_L(t)}{EMG_{L_{Max}}})$$

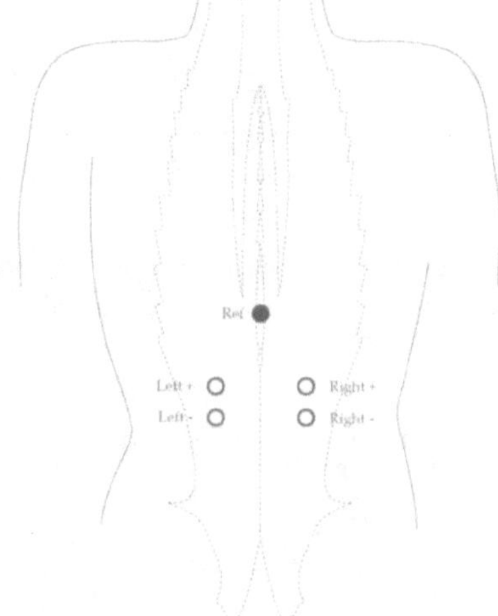

Figure 13: Electrode placement to acquire data from the erector spinae. Courtesy of [195]

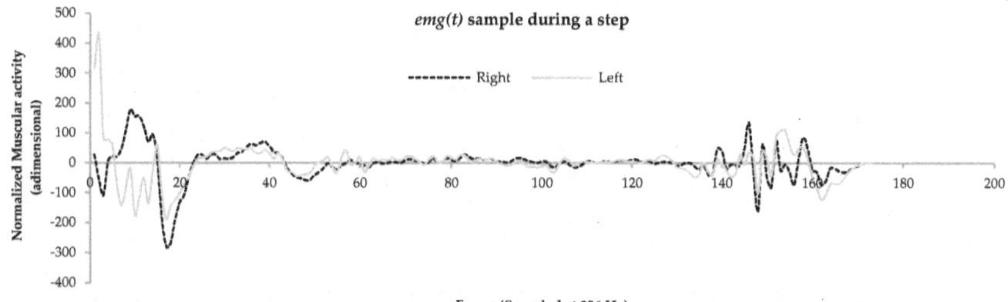

Figure 14: Electromyography sample during a step

The piezoelectric step sensor was placed directly under the heel of the dominant foot of the participant. It delivered a non-zero signal exclusively from the point the heel strikes on the floor ($t = heelstrike$) to the point where it is raised from the floor ($t = heeloff$). This sensor was used exclusively in the gait scenario, to mark the phases of the gait cycle (*Figure 15*). If we define $step(t)$ as the sensor value, $step(t = heelstrike)$ can be defined as the first non-zero value preceded by a zero, and heel off $step(t = heeloff)$ as the fist zero value preceded by a non-zero. We used this time values to calculate *HSMAX*, and *HOMAX* as described above.

$$t = heelstrike \leftrightarrow step(t) > 0, step(t-1) = 0,$$
$$t = heeloff \leftrightarrow step(t) > 0, step(t+1) = 0$$

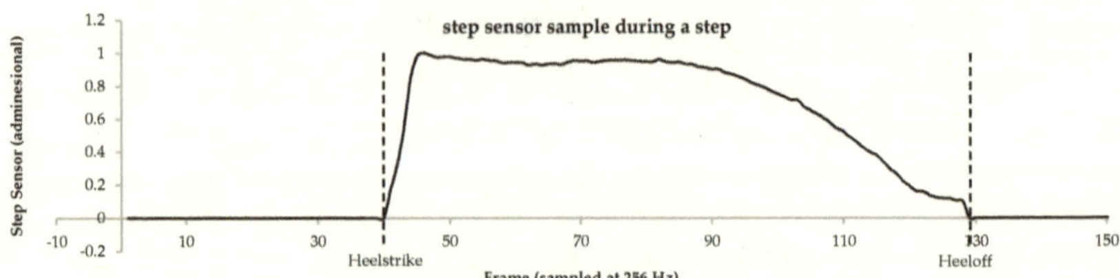

Figure 15: Step sensor sample during a step

Once all five data streams were acquired, synchronization was performed using cubic spline interpolation, to the timestamps of the force plate data. *Figure 16* describes the feature extraction process for both the standing and walking scenarios.

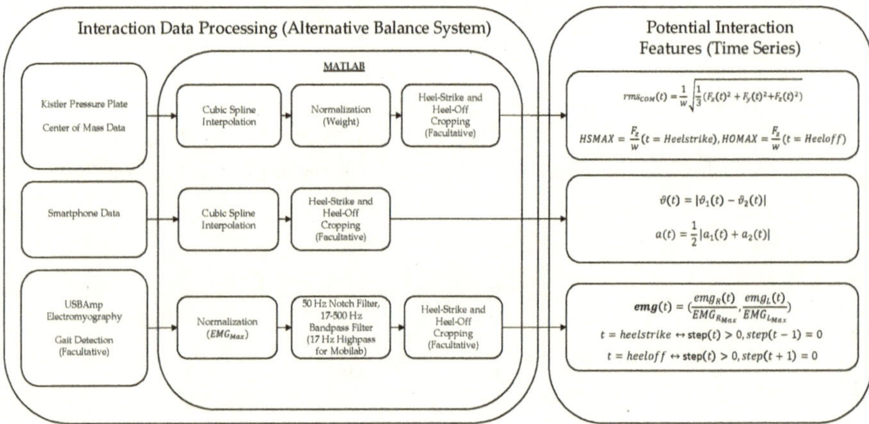

Figure 16: Alternative gait assessment system interaction data processing diagram

This approach was tested with a cohort of 40 participants (*Table 52*, median age 27, 18 males) split in a gait- and balance- affected group and an age- and sex-matched control group. The study was divided into two sections: (1) standing and (2) walking. In the standing section, participants stood over the pressure plate three times under three different conditions: with eyes open, with eyes closed and with eyes open standing on a foam pad. This test was thus performed a total of nine times, for 60 seconds per attempt. In the gait section, participants were asked to walk across a room in a straight line, with the pressure plate being in the middle. They were asked to walk at their preferred pace, and we ensured that they performed a full step over the pressure plate, without informing them as to not affect their gait. Due to data failure, two gait samples (one in the control and one in the intervention group) had to be removed. The test was repeated until we had three valid samples. From the time series described in *Figure 16*, we extracted the specific features included in *Table 9* for the standing scenario and *Table 10* for the walking scenario. We then attempted to train a classifier to discriminate if a participant belonged to the gait- and balance-affected group or was a healthy control, based on these features.

Features	Description	Calculation
$Rms_{COM\,Avg}$	Average of the rms_{COM} over the 60 second test, sampled at 1024 Hz, total sample number n_{RMSCOM}. Cubical spline interpolation. One value for each of the three tests, in three conditions, for a total of nine features	$\frac{\sum_{t=1}^{n_{RMSCOM}} rms_{COM}(t)}{n_{RMSCOM}}$
Emg_{Avg}	Average of the normalized muscular activity of the erector spinae over the 60 second sample, sampled at 1024 Hz, total sample number n_{EMG}. Two values (right, left) for each of the three tests, in three conditions, for a total of 18 features	$\frac{\sum_{t=1}^{n_{EMG}} \boldsymbol{emg}(t)}{n_{EMG}}$
$Rotation_{Avg}$	Average of the smartphone rotation values over the 60 second sample, sampled at 100 Hz, total sample number n_{ROT}. Cubical spline interpolation. One value for each of the three tests, in three conditions, for a total of nine features	$\frac{\sum_{t=1}^{t=n_{ROT}} \vartheta(t)}{n_{ROT}}$

Table 9: Alternative balance assessment system features for the standing scenario

Features	Description	Calculation
$HSMAX$	Vertical pressure plate force at $heelstrike$. One value for each of the three tests, for a total of three features	$\frac{F_z}{w}(t = heelstrike)$, $t = heelstrike \leftrightarrow step(t) > 0, step(t-1) = 0$
$HOMAX$	Vertical pressure plate force at $heeloff$. One value for each of the three tests, for a total of three features	$\frac{F_z}{w}(t = heeloff)$, $t = heeloff \leftrightarrow step(t) = 0, step(t+1) > 0$
Emg_{Avg}	Average of the normalized muscular activity of the erector spinae from heel-strike to heel-off, sampled at 256 Hz. Two values (right, left) for each of the three tests, for a total of six features	$\frac{\sum_{t=heelstrike}^{heeloff} \boldsymbol{emg}(t)}{heeloff - heelstrike}$
$Rotation_{Amp}$	Maximum amplitude of the rotation between heel-strike and heel-off. One value for each of the three tests, for a total of six features	$\max \vartheta(heelstrike, heeloff) - min\ \vartheta(heelstrike, heeloff)$
$Acceleration_{Std}$	Standard deviation of the forward acceleration between $heelstrike$ and $heeloff$. One value for each of the three tests, for a total of three features	$\sqrt{\frac{\sum_{t=heelstrike}^{heeloff}(a(t) - \bar{a})^2}{(heeloff - heelstrike) - 1}}$
N_{Steps}	Number of steps performed to cover the whole path. Counted as the number of non-zero regions in the step sensor data. One value for each of the three tests, for a total of three features	$N\ (step(t) > 0, t \neq heeloff)$

Table 10: Alternative balance assessment system features for the walking scenario

We found no statistically significant differences between groups, large effect sizes or successful classification methods in either scenario. For the standing scenario, classification results are included in *Table 11* and *Figure 17*, and statistical data are included in *Appendix E, Table 54*. For the walking scenario, classification results are provided in *Table 12* and *Figure 18*, and statistical data are provided in *Appendix E, Table 55*. Hyperparameters are described in *Appendix D, Table 50*. There are several possible reasons for these results. The complexity of bodily postural control may not be sufficiently described using only the employed data. Alternatively, it may be that the chosen tasks are not physically demanding enough to elicit differences in the features. Given these results, and considering that related studies with similar cohorts and goals did find significant differences when using the Wii Balance Board [70] we decided to use the Extended Balance Board for our implementation.

Algorithm: Multilayer Perceptron, accuracy 62.500%	Correctly classified	Incorrectly classified	TP rate	FP rate	Precision	F	MCC	ROC area	PRC area
Affected	14 (TP)	6 (FN)	0.700	0.450	0.609	0.651	0.253	0.580	0.585
Control	11 (TN)	9 (FP)	0.550	0.300	0.647	0.595	0.253	0.580	0.560
Weighted average	25	15	0.625	0.375	0.628	0.623	0.253	0.580	0.573
Algorithm: Decision Stump, accuracy 62.500%									
Affected	18 (TP)	2 (FN)	0.900	0.650	0.581	0.706	0.299	0.495	0.499
Control	7 (TN)	13 (FP)	0.350	0.100	0.778	0.483	0.299	0.495	0.580
Weighted average	25	15	0.625	0.375	0.679	0.594	0.299	0.495	0.540

Table 11: Alternative balance assessment system standing test classification results

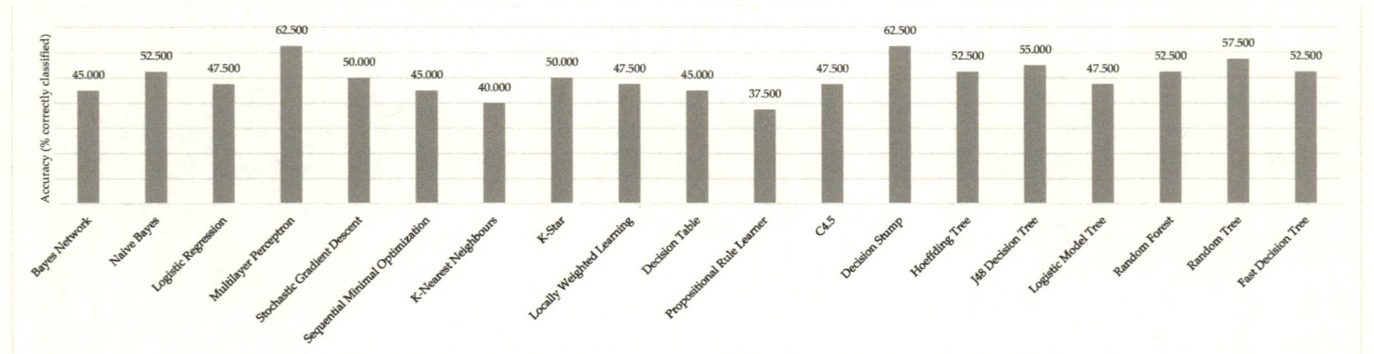

Figure 17: Alternative balance assessment system standing test classification accuracies

Algorithm: K-Nearest Neighbours, accuracy 52.632%	Correctly classified	Incorrectly classified	TP rate	FP rate	Precision	F	MCC	ROC area	PRC area
Affected	8 (TP)	11 (FN)	0.421	0.368	0.533	0.471	0.054	0.496	0.497
Control	12 (TN)	7 (FP)	0.632	0.579	0.522	0.571	0.054	0.496	0.500
Weighted average	20	18	0.526	0.474	0.528	0.521	0.054	0.496	0.498
Algorithm: J48 Decision Tree, accuracy 52.632%									
Affected	9	10	0.474	0.421	0.529	0.500	0.053	0.537	0.511
Control	11	8	0.579	0.526	0.524	0.550	0.053	0.537	0.540
Weighted average	20	18	0.526	0.474	0.527	0.525	0.053	0.537	0.526

Table 12: Alternative balance assessment system walking test classification results

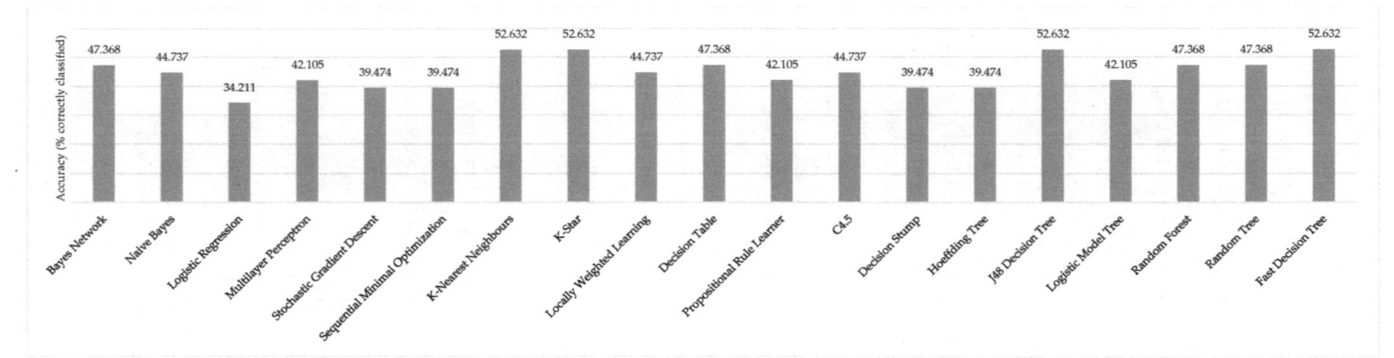

Figure 18: Alternative balance assessment system walking test classification accuracies

5.2. Exergame

Once a data acquisition system has been designed, an exergame was necessary to provide an engaging environment for data acquisition. In this case, the requirement was to design an exergame that included a cognitive task and a motor task, controlled with the Extended Balance Board. To achieve this goal, we designed PDDanceCity [91, 149, 272], with a cognitive task developed based on the results of previous work by Kalbe et al. [145]. PDDanceCity is a labyrinth game that presents the player with a randomly generated city map. The goal of the game is to navigate this map from a given starting point to a given goal, marked with a racing flag, by walking on the Extended Balance Board. The map is navigated using two-dimensional horizontal and vertical movements. Across the map, several waypoints (e.g., monuments) can be found, which the player may be asked to visit in a certain order, depending on difficulty. In addition, some streets can only be navigated in one direction (indicated by a directional arrow).

Based on factors relevant to cognitive tasks as described in [145], map generation is randomized from a series of variables (*Figure 19a*). The caregiver decides on a chart size (5x4, 6x5 or 7x6 elements), the presence of one-directional streets (none, few, several, many), the desired length of the optimal path (short, medium, long), and the number of waypoints (none, few, several, many). The caregiver can also decide whether certain elements will be only shown for a few seconds, and whether a step timer and/or metronome (to prevent freeze of gait) should be present. The step timer consists of auditory and visual cues in case a step is not taken after a number of seconds. The metronome is a ticking sound that can be adjusted in frequency. Once the map is created, a certain number of paths is removed, depending on map size and whether the edges can be navigated (*Figure 19b*). This removal is iterative. A path is selected randomly and, if there is another connection between the two edges, it is removed. The process is done this way to ensure all points can still be reached. If the removal would render a point inaccessible, another point is chosen instead. After element removal, one-way streets are added in the same process, again ensuring the complete map can be navigated (*Figure 19c*). The exact number of one-way streets depends on supervisor choice and map size.

Once the map is generated, the start and end points are placed (*Figure 19d*). This placement is based on the optimal path length choice, map size, and distribution, since the presence of many one-way streets may significantly lengthen the path. A minimum and maximum path length are calculated based on these parameters, and then a pair of points are chosen randomly. If the distance between these points falls within the minimum and maximum, they are set as start and end points. If not, two new points are chosen. If no points on the map fulfill these criteria, the map is discarded and the process begins again. In the final step, the waypoints are placed on the path (*Figure 19e*). The number of waypoints depends on map size. From the total number of waypoints to be placed, up to three are chosen and placed randomly within the optimal path. These are the waypoints to be visited. The rest are also placed randomly across the rest of the map.

Once the session begins, the character is positioned at the starting point. If a time limit is specified, this is shown on the lower right side of the screen. If the player has to pass through waypoints, these are shown on the left side of the screen. When a player reaches a waypoint, it is grayed out to visually show that the player has already visited that waypoint.

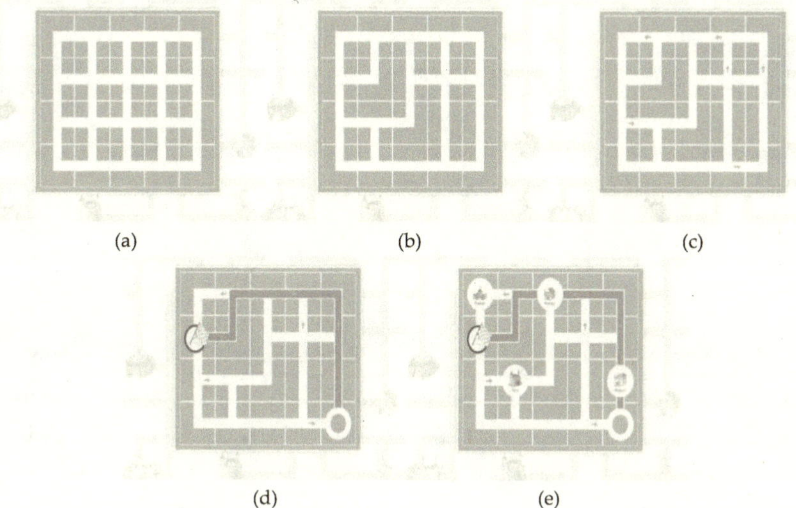

(a) (b) (c)

(d) (e)

Figure 19: PDDanceCity map generation process (left to right, and top to bottom), presented in [20]

During the game, several hints are displayed to support the player depending on the difficulty level. If the player reaches the goal before passing through all required waypoints, this is indicated. If the step timer runs out, a warning is also displayed. Finally, if the player attempts to enter a one-way street in the wrong direction, this is also indicated. Users are always encouraged to take the optimal path to their targets (marked by a red line) and the path they actually took is presented at the conclusion (as a blue line). After the user has reached the goal, they are presented with a questionnaire, in which the visited waypoints must be indicated. This section of the game is called quiz (*Figure 20*).

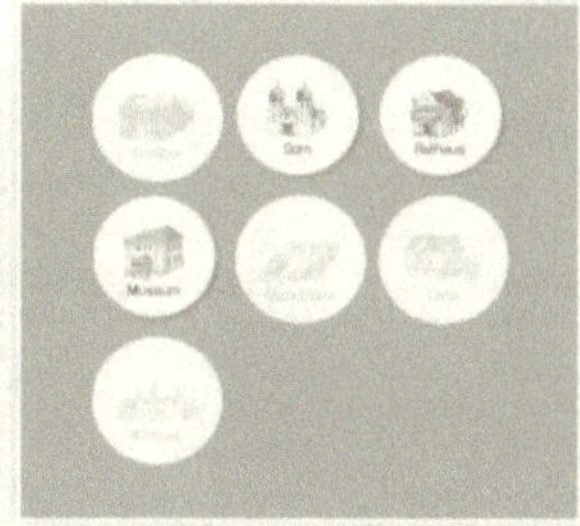

Figure 20: PDDanceCity quiz

The game offers varying levels of cognitive and motor difficulty. A higher cognitive difficulty has more one-directional streets, hides the goal after showing it for only a few seconds, and requests the user to visit a greater number of waypoints. A higher motor difficulty will cue the users to move faster, or require them to perform wider steps on the Extended Balance Board. A summary on the levels of cognitive and motor difficulty is presented in *Table 13*.

Cognitive difficulty levels	C1	C2	C3	C4	C5	C6
Start/End visible	Visible	Visible	Hidden	Visible	Visible	Hidden
Optimal path visible	Visible	Hidden	Hidden	Visible	Hidden	Hidden
Map size	Small	Medium	Large	Small	Medium	Large
One-way streets	None	Few	Many	None	Few	Many
Waypoints	None	None	None	Few	Many	All

Motor difficulty levels	M1	M2	M3	M1	M2	M3
Length of optimal path	Short	Medium	Long	Short	Medium	Long
Step timer	None	Long	Short	None	Long	Short

Table 13: PDDanceCity difficulty levels

The game combines cognitive and motor tasks. The cognitive task consists of mentally drawing a path in an urban environment, with disappearing goals, training both the visuospatial function and memory. The motor task consists of taking steps on a pressure plate. For each playthrough, the game data described in *Table 14* is acquired. This information includes the difficulty level played, the nature and number of cognitive errors (e.g., the waypoints were not identified correctly, the goal was not found, or the shortest path was not taken). It also includes the elapsed time, the time between steps and the relation between the number of steps performed and the minimum steps required to reach the goal.

Features	Description	Features	Description
Cognitive difficulty	Cognitive difficulty level of the session (*Table 13*)	Path game tries	Final goal not found or waypoint ignored
Motor difficulty	Motor difficulty level of the session (*Table 13*)	Target game tries	Number of times where a player states that a target was found, but the target has not been reached yet
Quiz errors	Number of errors in the quiz	Number of steps and shortest path differential	Total number of steps, difference in steps between path taken and optimal path
One-way errors	Number of attempts to walk in a one-directional street in the wrong direction	Total time	Total playthrough time
Motivity errors	Number of attempts to take steps in nonexisting directions (walls)	Time per step	Time elapsed between each step
Motivity timer expired	Number of times the step timer expired without input	Map data	Map size, number of one-way streets and waypoints

Table 14: PDDanceCity game data features

5.3. Evaluation

Cohort and Study Design

The evaluation of this clinical decision support system should determine its accuracy in assessing the risk of falling. We decided to test the accuracy of the system in its capacity to perform a binary fall risk classification (average risk and increased risk) when compared to a clinical gold standard.

For this evaluation, we use the 30-Second-Sit-To-Stand Test [270] as our clinical outcome. We chose this test for its excellent test-retest and interrater reliability [141]. It is a measure of lower extremity strength in older adults and is part of the Fullerton Fitness Test Battery. The test is performed as follows. The participant begins sitting on a chair without arms. The chair is fixed in place (i.e. set against a wall). Participants sit, with their back straight and their feet completely on the floor at approximately shoulder width. In order to improve balance, one leg may be slightly more extended than the other. The participant is then asked to stand up, and sit back down fully, without using their arms, as many times as possible for thirty seconds ensuring balance is not lost. Each correct repetition adds one point, but if the patient uses their arms at any moment, they are scored zero points. The evaluator may visually perform the task or ask the participant to try it once to clarify, prior to administering the test. The cutoff scores to indicate the capability of maintaining physical independence are age-dependent. For example, cutoff scores are 15 for females and 17 for males aged 60-64 and 9 for both males and females aged 90 or older. The goal of our system is to perform a binary prediction of the result of this test by collecting data from the Extended Balance Board while playing PDDanceCity. The complete system diagram, as conceived in *Chapter 4*, is depicted in *Figure 21*. The list of employed features is included in *Table 15*.

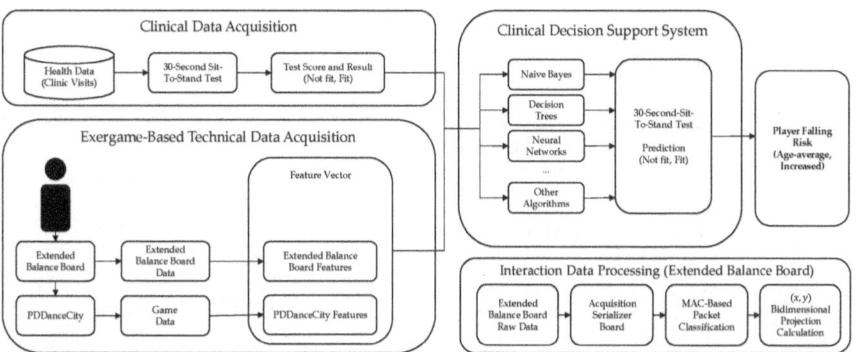

Figure 21: Exergame-based clinical decision support system to assess balance. System diagram

Features	Description	Calculation
$Com_{Avg_{Direction}}$	Average **com** value for upwards, downwards, rightwards and leftwards movements, where $n_{COM,Direction}$ is the number of steps in each direction. Four two-dimensional features (x, y) per playthrough	$\frac{\sum_{t=1}^{n_{COM,Direction}} com(t)}{n_{COM,Direction}}$ $Direction = Up \leftrightarrow com_y > 0.5, \lvert com_x \rvert < 0.1$ $Direction = Down \leftrightarrow com_y < -0.5, \lvert com_x \rvert < 0.1$ $Direction = Right \leftrightarrow com_x > 0.5, \lvert com_y \rvert < 0.1$ $Direction = Left \leftrightarrow com_x < -0.5, \lvert com_y \rvert < 0.1$
$Com_{Std_{Direction}}$	Standard deviation of **com,** per direction, as above. Eight features per playthrough	$\sqrt{\frac{\sum_{t=1}^{n_{COM,Direction}} \left(com_i(t) - Com_{Avg_{Direction,i}}\right)^2}{n_{COM,j} - 1}}$, $i = x, y, Direction = Up, Down, Left, Right$
$Balance_{Up}$, $Balance_{Down}$	Average value of com_y for all values where $com_y > 0$ (up) or $com_y < 0$ (down) and n_{COM} is the total number of **com** samples. Two features per playthrough	$\frac{\sum_{t=1}^{n_{COM}} com_y(t)}{n_{COM}} : com_y > 0, \frac{\sum_{t=1}^{n_{COM}} com_y(t)}{n_{COM}} : com_y < 0$
$Balance_{Right}$, $Balance_{Left}$	Average value of com_x for all values where $com_x > 0$ (right) or $com_x < 0$ (left). Two features per playthrough	$\frac{\sum_{t=1}^{n_{COM}} com_x(t)}{n_{COM}} : com_x > 0, \frac{\sum_{t=1}^{n_{COM}} com_x(t)}{n_{COM}} : com_x < 0$
Avg_x, Avg_y	Average value of com_x and com_y. Two features (x, y) per playthrough	$\frac{\sum_{t=1}^{n_{COM}} com_x(t)}{n_{COM}}, \frac{\sum_{t=1}^{n_{COM}} com_y(t)}{n_{COM}}$
Max_x, Max_y, Min_x, Min_y	Maximum and minimum value of com_x and com_y. Four features per playthrough	$Max\ (com_x(t), \forall t), Max\ (com_y(t), \forall t)$, $Min\ (com_x(t), \forall t), Max\ (com_y(t), \forall t)$
Std_x, Std_y	Standard deviation of com_x and com_y. Two features (x, y) per playthrough	$\sqrt{\frac{\sum_{t=1}^{n_{COM}} (com_i(t) - Avg_i)^2}{n_{COM} - 1}}, i = x, y$
If_{Avg}, If_{Max}	Average $if(t)$ value and maximum for the whole playthrough. Two features per playthrough	$\frac{\sum_{t=1}^{n_{COM}} if(t)}{n_{COM}}, Max\ (if(t), \forall t)$
$If_{Threshold,i}$	Number of times $if(t) > i, i = [0.5,1,1.5,2]$. Normalized by total playthrough time. Four features per playthrough	$\frac{N\ (if(t) > i)}{n_{COM}}, i = 0.5,1,1.5,2$
$If_{Sum_{Avg}}$, $If_{Sum_{Max}}$	Average value and maximum of the sum of the last 25 values of $if(t)$ for the whole playthrough. Two features per playthrough	$\frac{\sum_{t=1}^{n_{COM}} if_{Sum}(t)}{n_{COM}}, if_{Sum}(t) = \sum_{i=t-24}^{t} if(t)$, $Max\ (if_{Sum}(t), \forall t)$
$If_{Sum_{Overx}}$	Number of times $If_{Sum}(t) > i, i = [0.5,1,1.5,2]$. Normalized by total playthrough time. Four features per playthrough	$\frac{N\ (if_{Sum}(t) > i)}{n_{COM}}, i = 0.5,1,1.5,2$
$Step_{Avg}$	Average time between steps, excluding the first step, defining $Step_{Time}(i)$ as the time in seconds in which step i occurred, and n_{Steps} as the total number of steps in the playthrough. One feature per playthrough	$\frac{\sum_{i=2}^{n_{Steps}} Step_{Time}(i) - Step_{Time}(i-1)}{n_{Steps}}$
$Step_{Std}$	Standard deviation of time between steps, excluding the first step. One feature per playthrough	$\sqrt{\frac{\sum_{i=2}^{n_{Steps}} \left(Step_{Time}(i) - Step_{Time}(i-1) - Step_{Avg}\right)^2}{n_{Steps} - 1}}$
Age, Sex	Player-related nominal data: age and sex. Two features per playthrough	

Table 15: Exergame-based clinical decision support system to assess balance. System features

For this test, a cohort of 16 participants (*Table 52,* median age 73, 6 males) were selected and recruited from a nursing home in Darmstadt. There were no specific inclusion criteria, considering the nursing home would provide participants adequate for the evaluation. The exclusion criterion was severe balance impairment that could implicate a serious risk of falling during the evaluation, judged by a physiotherapist. Two of the participants had dementia, and one had PD. 67% of participants declared little or no experience with computers. During the first session, participants were asked to perform the 30-Second-Sit-to-Stand Test. Personal information (age, sex) was collected. Afterwards, they played a level of PDDanceCity with supervision. A user profile was created in the game. For further sessions, participants chose their profile, played as long as they wanted, and then left. An evaluator was present to ensure participants did not fall from the device, but otherwise the remaining playthroughs were unsupervised. A total of 87 levels of PDDanceCity were played, of which 6 were discarded due to data failure, leaving a dataset of 16 participants and 81 playthroughs. All participants started at the lowest difficulty level of PDDanceCity (C1,M1, see *Table 13*) and the difficulty was subsequently increased if performance was satisfactory and the player agreed. This increase occurred either at the suggestion of the player or the evaluator. Difficulty was always increased on a step-to-step basis.

For the purpose of this evaluation we consider two evaluation scenarios, considering that the cutoff scores of the Sit-To-Stand test are age-dependent. First, we design a classification scenario without player-related nominal data. In this scenario, we consider players are fit if they score 12 points or higher in the Sit-To-Stand test. The results of this scenario are presented in *Table 16* and *Figure 22*. For the second scenario, we include age and sex as classification features, and distribute participants as fit or not fit depending on the age- and sex-adjusted cutoff scores described in the Sit-To-Stand test instructions. This means that a participant may be classified as "fit" for the first scenario and "not fit" for the second, but this was only the case with three participants). The results of this scenario are included in *Table 17* and *Figure 23*. The age- and sex-adjusted cutoff scores, as well as statistical details on both classification scenarios are provided in *Appendix E,* section *Extended Balance Board Evaluation Classification Results*.

Results

Classification results are good in both cases. In short, it is possible to predict whether the user will score below, or above, 12 points on the sit-to-stand test based on data collected by playing PDDanceCity. If the player is known, predicting the result of the test, with an age- and sex-adjusted cutoff score is also possible. Effect sizes of features, presented in *Appendix E, Table 57* and *Table 58,* indicate the most relevant features are those related to the instability factor $if(t)$ and to the mean time and standard deviation of steps $Step_{Avg}$, $Step_{Std}$. Effect sizes seem to be larger in the scenario with nominal data, but in both cases the largest effect sizes are achieved on $if(t)$ features. Classifier hyperparameters are provided in *Appendix D, Table 50*. The quality of these results is increased by the nature of the evaluation scenario. Since participants did not need supervision, a home-based scenario seems to be feasible as long as the Extended Balance Board can be placed in a position where the risk of falling backwards is completely eliminated (i.e. against a wall). The main limitation for this potential scenario is the board setup process. At the moment, at first setup, the Wii Balance Boards need to be synchronized via Bluetooth with the Acquisition Serializer Board. This connection then remains active until the device runs out of batteries, which usually takes approximately two days of continuous operation. A completely automatic setup process, combined with adapting the boards to operate with externally provided electrical power, would ensure the potential home-based scenario is indeed feasible.

Algorithm: Logistic Model Tree, accuracy 91.358%	Correctly classified	Incorrectly classified	TP rate	FP rate	Precision	F	MCC	ROC area	PRC area
Not fit	29 (TP)	5 (FN)	0.853	0.043	0.935	0.892	0.823	0.940	0.946
Fit	45 (TN)	2 (FP)	0.957	0.147	0.900	0.928	0.823	0.940	0.930
Weighted average	74	7	0.914	0.103	0.915	0.913	0.823	0.940	0.936
Algorithm: Fast Decision Tree, accuracy 87.654%									
Not fit	27 (TP)	7 (FN)	0.794	0.064	0.900	0.844	0.746	0.853	0.858
Fit	44 (TN)	3 (FP)	0.936	0.206	0.863	0.898	0.746	0.853	0.844
Weighted average	71	10	0.877	0.146	0.878	0.875	0.746	0.853	0.850

Table 16: Extended Balance Board classification results without player nominal data

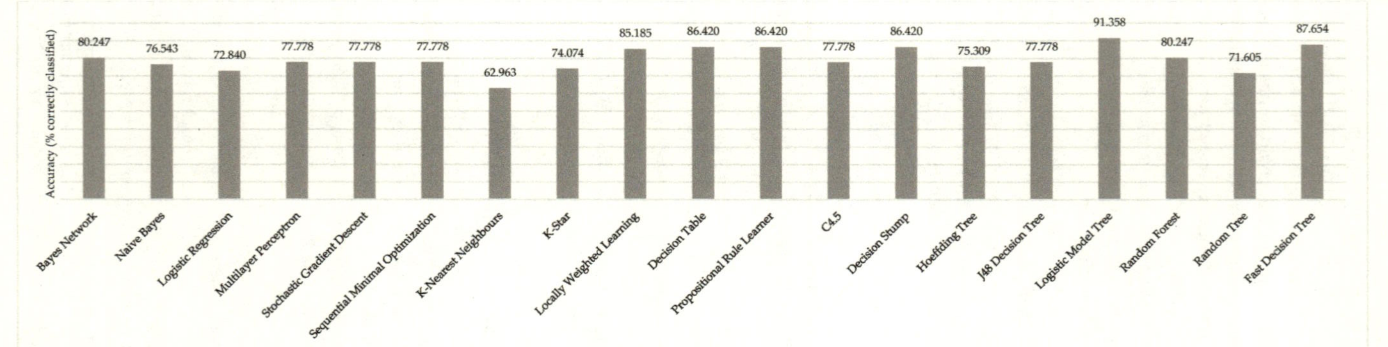

Figure 22: Extended Balance Board classification accuracies without player nominal data

Algorithm: C4.5, accuracy 98.765%	Correctly classified	Incorrectly classified	TP rate	FP rate	Precision	F	MCC	ROC area	PRC area
Not fit	35 (TP)	0 (FN)	1	0.022	0.972	0.986	0.975	0.989	0.972
Fit	45 (TN)	1 (FP)	0.978	0	1	0.989	0.975	0.989	0.991
Weighted average	80	1	0.988	0.009	0.988	0.988	0.975	0.989	0.983
Algorithm: Logistic Model Tree, accuracy 98.765%									
Not fit	34 (TP)	1 (FN)	0.971	0	1	0.986	0.975	1	1
Fit	46 (TN)	0 (FP)	1	0.029	0.979	0.989	0.975	1	1
Weighted average	80	1	0.988	0.016	0.988	0.988	0.975	1	1

Table 17: Extended Balance Board classification results with player nominal data

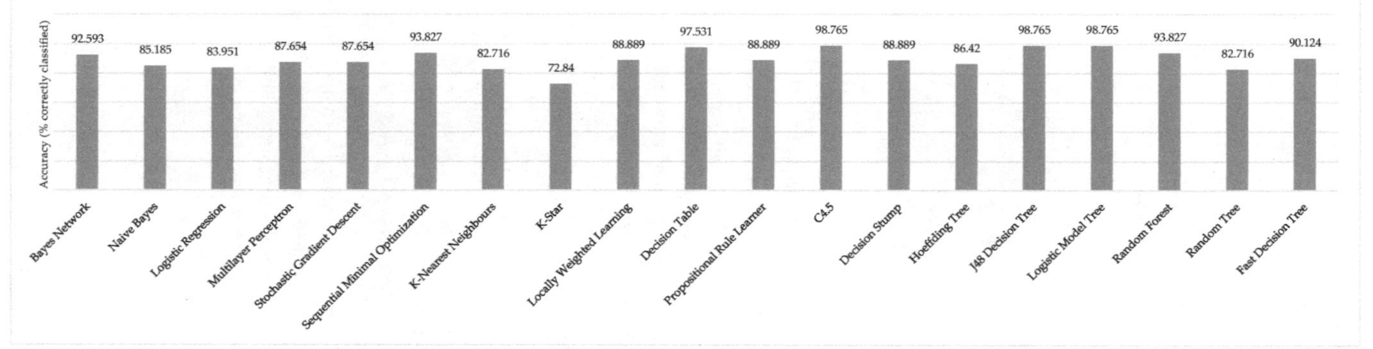

Figure 23: Extended Balance Board classification accuracies with player nominal data

Feature	Effect Size (g) without nominal data	Effect size (g) with nominal data
$Balance_{Left}$	0.6306	0.8976
Std_x	-0.6665	-1.2422
If_{Avg}	-0.7478	-2.0057
If_{Max}	-0.6337	-1.2166
$If_{Threshold,0.}$	-0.7452	-1.4445
$If_{Sum_{Avg}}$	-0.7387	-1.9909
$If_{Sum_{Over\ 0.5}}$	-1.5261	-2.0229
$If_{Sum_{Over\ 1}}$	-0.9196	-1.8100
$Step_{Avg}$	1.2260	1.0735
$Step_{Std}$	0.8446	0.8934

Table 18: Extended balance board classification results. Effect sizes of statistically significant features in both scenarios

PDDanceCity Acceptance

The acceptance of PDDanceCity was tested twice: once with the 16 participants of the balance and gait evaluation, and once separately with 28 healthy individuals of any age, in a study organized by the University Hospital Cologne. These 44 participants were asked to give their opinion on the game with two questions that could be answered on a one (disagree) to four (agree) Likert scale, regarding fun and user-friendliness. The 16 participants of the balance and gait evaluation also replied to two additional questions regarding skill adjustment and a potential home scenario use, since they would be the target population of a home scenario implementation.

In general terms, users found the game to be intuitive and user-friendly. Most users found the difficulty to be adequate to their skill. Participants with chronic diseases (PD and dementia) could still interact with the game properly. As displayed in *Figure 24*, user ratings were good for both fun and user-friendliness. On the other hand, the prospect of playing the game at home by themselves was rated slightly worse, as shown in *Figure 25*. Although most players found the difficulty level to be well-adjusted, only 66% of participants would play the game by themselves at home. Verbally, users reported that the latency between the Extended Balance Board and the game was too high, and that it did not always detect steps correctly. In summary, acceptance results are quite positive in all fields except the possibility of playing the game at home, which shows potential for improvement. A discussion on potential future work based on the results of the evaluation and user acceptance is presented in *Chapter 9*.

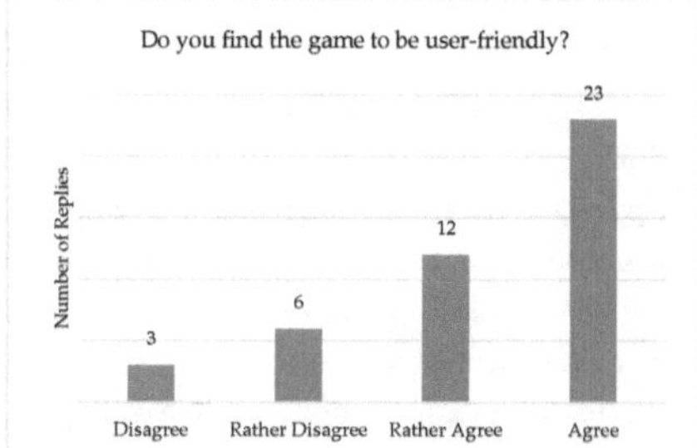

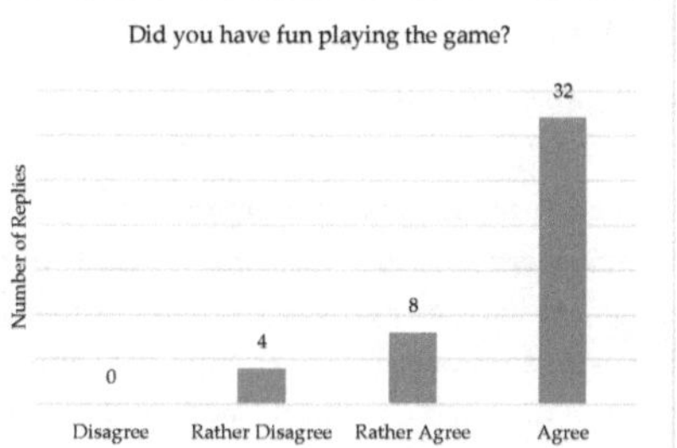

Figure 24: PDDanceCity acceptance test results for user-friendliness and fun

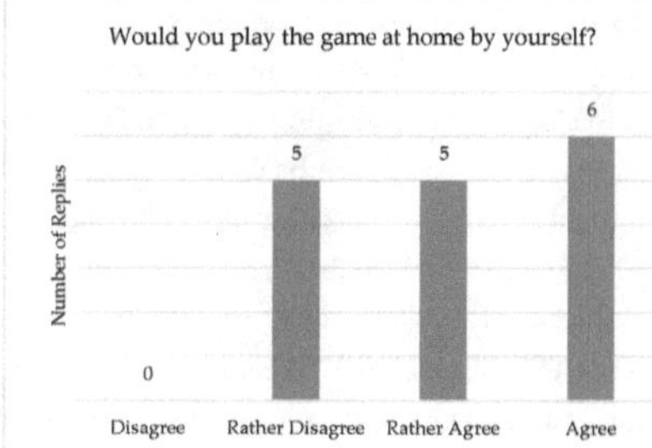

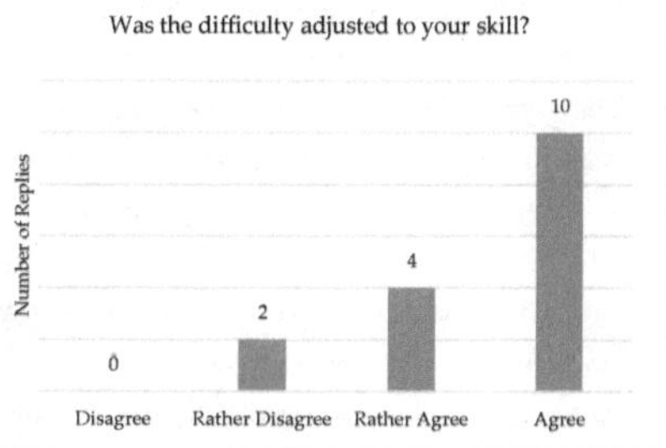

Figure 25: PDDanceCity acceptance test results for home monitoring potential and skill adjustment

6. Design of an Exergame-based Clinical Decision Support System to Assess Tremor

Based on our model for an exergame-based clinical decision support system to monitor a symptom of PD introduced in *Chapter 4*, in this chapter, we present a proof of concept of this model to assess hand tremor and hand dexterity. First, we describe the sensor that we used to control our system, the Leap Motion sensor. A number of alternatives were considered, as described in the section *Assessing Resting Tremor* of *Chapter 3*. However, the Leap Motion sensor presents an important advantage compared to these options, since it can be used to evaluate both hand tremor and bradykinesia, as discussed in *Chapter 3*. This is also possible with electromyography, but the Leap Motion sensor is non-invasive, which means that a potential home scenario is possible. We used the Leap Motion Sensor to implement a digitalized version of the current clinical standard to assess hand tremor and dexterity, Section III of the UPDRS test. We refer to this implementation as PALM (Parkinson Assessment with Leap Motion) [99]. The goal of PALM is to use the Leap Motion sensor to objectively determine parameters obtained from hand movements (e.g., speeds and amplitudes) which can be used as a basis to predict UPDRS scores. After concluding this design, we created a dual-tasking exergame controlled with the Leap Motion sensor, called PDPuzzleTable. This exergame, published in [93], is a series of digitalized puzzles that can provide data related to the player's cognitive skills based on game data, and obtain the same hand movement information as collected in PALM. In a preliminary test, we evaluated the capacity of the Leap Motion sensor to accurately discriminate a group of five PD patients and five healthy controls based on PALM features that evaluate resting tremor and bradykinesia [99]. Our results indicate that the system can accurately classify PD patients and healthy controls. Experimental details of this evaluation are provided in *Appendix F*. We conclude this chapter with an acceptance test of PDPuzzleTable. In this test, we studied the opinion of users and measured their performance when interacting with the sensor. Potential users found the game to be user-friendly and fun. However, we observed a significant learning effect when using the Leap Motion sensor, which has to be taken into consideration.

6.1. Data Acquisition

The Leap Motion sensor is a device capable of identifying hands and tracking finger movements individually with two infrared cameras and three infrared LEDs. It has a surface of 3-by-8 cm, with a height of 1.25 cm. The LEDs generate infrared light and the cameras capture reflected data at a frequency of up to 200 Hz. Proprietary machine learning algorithms, running on the computer, then detect the position of different parts of the hand, with a positional error of approximately 0.7 mm (*Figure 26*) [164]. It is possible to obtain the data produced by these proprietary algorithms by using the LeapC library [320]. We refer to these data as our raw data (*Table 19*).

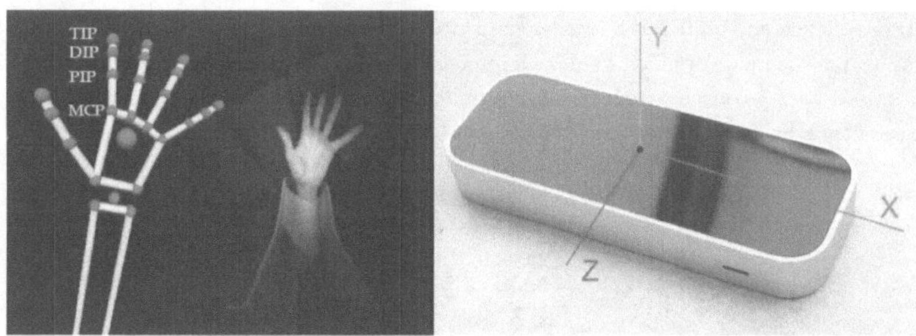

Figure 26: Leap Motion hand recognition (left), sensor and coordinate system (right). The four tracking points per finger, as described in *Table 19*, are indicated for the index finger

Parameter	Name	Description
Hand ID	hand_id	Hand unique identifier (several hands can be detected at the same time)
Hand type	type	Hand type (left/right)
Hand palm center	palm_position	Cartesian coordinates (x, y, z) of the center of the palm in mm (see *Figure 26*)
Hand palm rotation	palm_normal	Cartesian coordinates (x, y, z) of a vector perpendicular to the palm, pointing downwards
Wrist position	wrist	Cartesian coordinates (x, y, z) of the wrist of the hand
Finger type	finger_id	Finger type (0 to 4, 0 being the thumb and 4 the index finger)
Finger metacarpophalangeal joint position	mcp_position	Cartesian coordinates (x, y, z) of the metacarpophalangeal joint, per finger (see *Figure 26)*
Finger proximal interphalangeal joint position	pip_position	Cartesian coordinates (x, y, z) of the proximal interphalangeal joint, per finger (see *Figure 26)*
Finger distal interphalangeal joint position	dip_position	Cartesian coordinates (x, y, z) of the distal interphalangeal joint, per finger (see *Figure 26)*
Fingertip position	tip_position	Cartesian coordinates (x, y, z) of the fingertip, per finger (see *Figure 26)*
Finger width	width	Estimated finger width in mm, per finger
Finger length	length	Estimated finger length in mm, per finger
Pinch strength	pinch_strength	Adimensional value 0-1 (0 for open hand, 1 for closed pinch)
Grab strength	grab_strength	Adimensional value 0-1 (0 for open hand, 1 for closed fist)
Grab angle	grab_angle	Angle between fingers and grabbing hand pose (0 for open hand, pi for closed fist)

Table 19: Leap Motion sensor raw data [320]

The Leap Motion sensor offers three different resolutions: high speed (low resolution), balanced, and high precision (high resolution). We used the balanced option as indicated by previous authors [42]. In order to improve the accuracy of the data acquisition process, an armature such as the one presented in [9] was designed and built. It is a wooden structure with a surface of 22-by-41 cm, and a height of 29 cm. The arm rest is made of fabric to make it more comfortable. We included an improvement in our design: the sensor lays on a movable tray to ensure it is always placed under the hand (*Figure 27*). This has to be taken into consideration since PD patients have limited hand mobility.

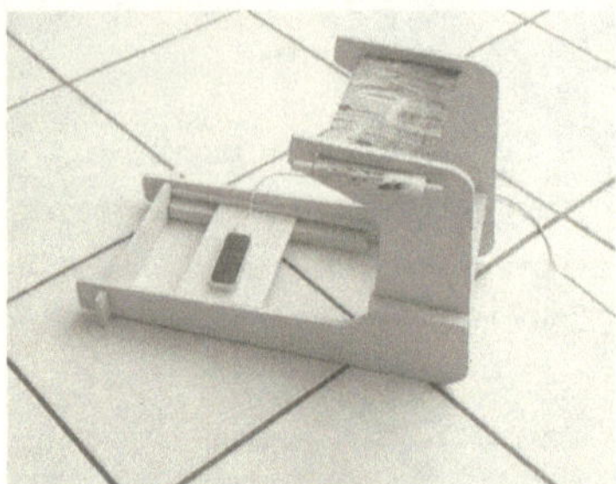

Figure 27: Leap Motion armature

Once we could acquire raw hand movement data from the Leap Motion sensor, our next task was to implement a data acquisition procedure. The state of PD patients is regularly evaluated by their neurologists using the UPDRS test [108]. This test evaluates numerous aspects of the PD patient, one of which is their hand dexterity (UPDRS Tasks 3.4 to 3.6) and tremor (UPDRS Tasks 3.15 and 3.16). These tasks are described as follows:

- **UPDRS III Task 3.4: Finger Tapping.** The patient should tap the index finger on the thumb ten times, as quickly and widely as possible. The task should be performed with both hands, which should be rated separately.
- **UPDRS III Task 3.5: Hand Movements.** The patient should open and close their hand, forming a fist, ten times, as quickly and widely as possible. The tasked should be performed with both hands, which should be rated separately. In order to avoid confusion, in this document this task will be henceforth referred to as **Fist Closing**.
- **UPDRS III Task 3.6: Pronation-Supination of Hands.** The patient should turn the palm up and down alternately, ten times, as quickly and widely as possible. The task should be performed with both hands, which should be rated separately.
- **UPDRS III Task 3.15: Postural Tremor.** The patient should stretch their arms in front of the body with the palms down. The fingers should be comfortably separated. Observe the tremor amplitude in this posture for ten seconds.
- **UPDRS III Task 3.16: Kinetic Tremor.** The patient should perform three finger-to-nose maneuvers with each hand reaching as far as possible to touch the examiner's finger. Observe the highest tremor amplitude seen.

Exercises are then rated on a scale of zero (no symptoms) to four (unable to perform the task). Although guidelines for scores are provided, these evaluations have a margin for subjectivity. The guidelines of Tasks 3.4 to 3.6 discuss speed, acceleration, interruptions, and amplitudes. The neurologist is required to evaluate all these factors visually and simultaneously. In Tasks 3.15 and 3.16, the neurologist is required to distinguish a tremor with an amplitude of two cm from another with an amplitude of four.

These factors may cause two neurologists to rate the same PD patient differently. Further details on these tasks is provided in *Appendix A*, *Table 37* and *Table 38*.

We decided to implement a digitalized version of the UPDRS test using the Leap Motion sensor. As described in *Table 19*, the sensor can provide information related to all of the aspects that have to be considered to rate the UPDRS tasks. For this purpose, we created PALM (Parkinson Assessment with Leap Motion). PALM is an application where the hand, as recognized by the sensor, is visually presented to ensure data are being acquired correctly. PALM collects the raw data described in *Table 19* in the background, and extracts relevant classification features using a series of Matlab algorithms.

In collaboration with physiotherapists as well as doctors, a system was implemented in which a total of five tasks are performed, in extension of the UPDRS tasks (*Table 20*).

PALM task	Related UPDRS task	Description
1. Static hand test	3.15	The patient should rest their hand on the armature, with extended, comfortably separated fingers, and hold still for 60 seconds. This task is performed once for each hand
2. Finger tapping	3.4, 3.16	The patient should rest their hand on the armature and tap the index finger on the thumb ten times, as quickly and widely as possible. The task is performed once for each hand
3. First closing	3.5, 3.16	The patient should rest their hand on the armature and open and close their hand, forming a fist, ten times, as quickly and widely as possible. The task is performed once for each hand
4. Pronation-supination	3.6, 3.16	The patient should rest their hand on the armature and turn the palm up and down alternately, ten times, as quickly and widely as possible. The task is performed once per hand
5. Lateral movement	3.16	The patient should rest their hand on the armature and position their hand as if they were holding a glass, laterally move their wrist left and right, ten times, as quickly and widely as possible. The task is performed once per hand

Table 20: Description of PALM Tasks

Once the tasks are performed, data are then processed using a series of algorithms programmed in Matlab. Essentially, PALM extracts the relevant data from each sample depending on which task was performed, and obtains a series of features which set the base for an assessment score by a neurologist, or for machine learning-based UPDRS score prediction (*Figure 28*).

For each task, PALM extracts features relevant to the related UPDRS task criteria from one or several of the signals described in *Table 19*. For example, for the static hand test (Task 1), we consider the maximum tremor amplitude of the palm center, as described in UPDRS Task 3.15. In general terms, we extract time-domain (amplitude, means, standard deviations) and frequency-domain features based on the Fast Fourier Transformation (FFT) in each task. In those that include a voluntary action (Tasks 2 to 5), we also include features related to the speed and amplitude with which this action was performed. We refer to these as kinetic features. A diagram describing the system is presented in *Figure 28*. Kinetic feature extraction is described in the section *Kinetic Signal Processing*. A description of each task, and the specific features considered in each task follows in the section *PALM Task Description*.

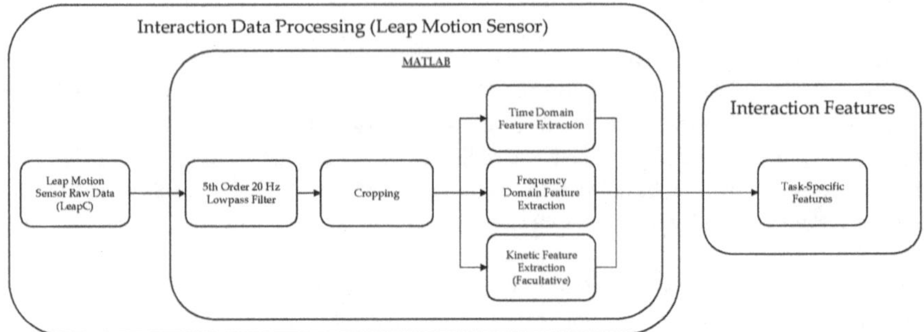

Figure 28: PALM interaction data processing diagram

Kinetic Signal Processing

In kinetic signals, the goal is to extract relevant features for amplitude and speed related to possible dexterity affections (e.g., interruptions, reductions in amplitude, or kinetic tremor). Signals recorded from an active task (PALM Tasks 2 to 5, *Table 20*) need to be cropped to the specific segment in which the task occurs. Afterwards, the points of interest have to be identified. This is done by using a combination of peak and zero-crossing detection algorithms in several iterations, and works as follows: let $s(t)$ be the position of the point of interest of the hand, as described in *Table 19* using the coordinate system depicted in *Figure 26*. Let $v(t)$ be speed of the same point of interest, calculated as the first order differential of $s(t)$, that is:

$$v(t) = s(t) - s(t-1), \nexists\, t' : t > t' > t-1$$

Then the signal is cropped as follows:

- Relative maxima of $|v(t)|$ are identified with a range of ± 0.25 seconds. This means that if the speed in this point is equal or greater than all values in this range, it is identified as a maximum. This range ensures that all relevant maxima are detected.

- All maxima with a value lesser or equal than 2.5 mm/s are set to zero, since such low speeds are not indicative of a voluntary movement.

- Each non-zero preceded by at least four zeros (that is, one second) is a potential start. If no potential start is found, the start of the signal is considered instead.

- Each non-zero followed by at least four zeros (that is, one second) is a potential end. If no potential end is found, the end of the signal is considered.

- The number of oscillations between each start and each end are calculated using zero-crossing detection. If a combination of a start and end contains ten oscillations, the signal is cropped to this range. If only combinations with more than ten oscillations are found, we crop a segment of that range that contains ten oscillations by counting zero crossings. If only combinations with less than ten oscillations are found, the combination with the greatest number of oscillations is taken. *Figure 29* depicts the cropping process.

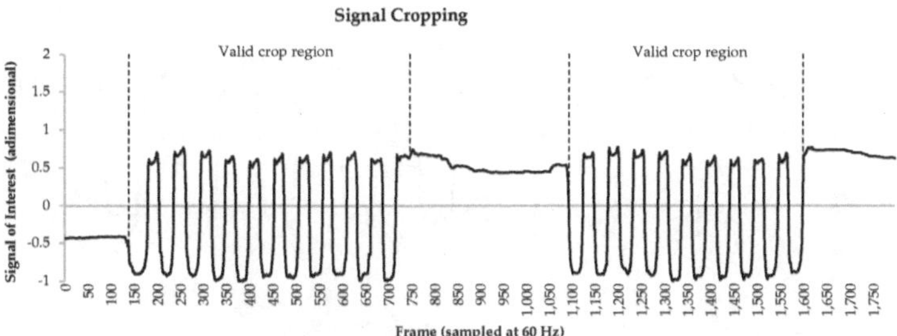

Figure 29: Kinetic cropping example. Two valid regions are detected, but the one on the left has ten oscillations and is preferable.

Once the signal has been cropped, the signal is processed. In the processing phase, we analyze the signal and detect the points of interest. This works as follows:

- Relative maxima and minima are identified in $s(t)$ with a comparison range of ± 0.25 seconds. This produces a vector of maxima (x, y), namely $\max(s(t))$ and a vector of minima (x, y), namely $\min(s(t))$.

- Tremor peaks (false peaks) are then removed: if a maximum has a value that is $\pm 30\%$ the average value of all minima, it is removed. The same procedure is then carried out with the minima.

- Finally, a peak correction procedure is performed in case the previous step removed a real maximum or minimum. In case no maximum is found between two minima, or no minimum is found between two maxima, a new one is added by finding the absolute maximum (or minimum) in the region where there should be one. This is necessary for signals where the tremor is very significant.

Once cropped and preprocessed, the following kinetic features are extracted:

- Amplitude related features: amplitudes are measured as the difference between each maximum and its successive minimum. Since analysis takes place between the first and last maxima, if n repetitions are performed, $n - 1$ amplitudes are extracted.

- Speed related features: hand speed has its maximum at the middle of the opening or closing movement. The points of interest are the maxima, as well as the first and last zero of the speed. For example, in an opening movement, the speed signal is a series of zeros (the hand is closed), followed by a number of non-zeros with a maximum (opening movement) followed by a series of zeros again (the hand is open). This allows us to measure both the opening speed and time, as well as the amount of time that the hand was opened or closed. Since the analysis takes place between the first and last maxima, if n repetitions are performed, $n-2$ speed-related features are extracted. This procedure is depicted in *Figure 30.*

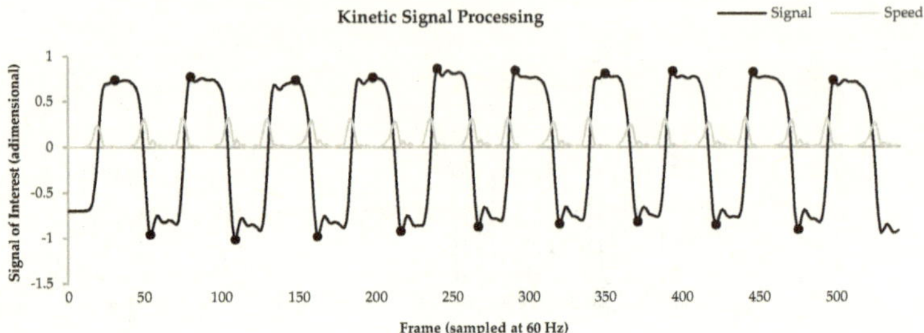

Figure 30: Kinetic processing example. Amplitudes are calculated on the basis of the maxima and minima, marked as dots. Zero regions of the speed are employed as open and closed hand periods

PALM Task Description and Features

Task 1: Static Hand Test

The goal of Task 1 (*Figure 31*) is to detect resting hand tremor. Given that the Leap Motion sensor refresh rate is variable (approximately 60 to 200 Hz, depending on ambient light and processing power), a sample length of 60 seconds was decided upon. The average framerate is calculated for each sample and taken into account when calculating time- and frequency-domain features.

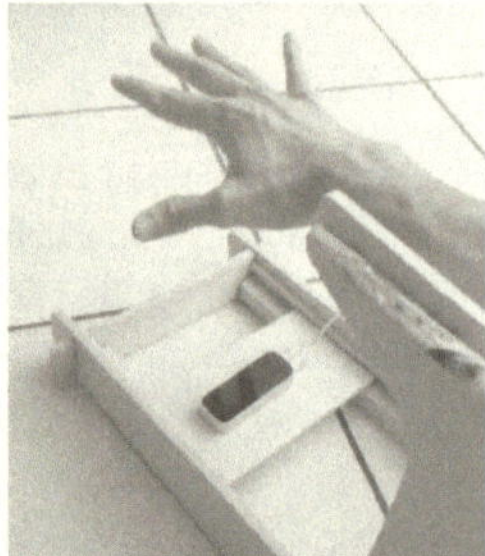

Figure 31: PALM Task 1

For this task, the signal of interest is the x cartesian coordinate of the palm center of the hand, that is:

$$s(t) = palm_{position_x}(t)$$

The coordinate is described in *Table 19* and the resulting signal is depicted in *Figure 32*. This signal was chosen because, after sampling numerous PD patients, we noticed tremor is most visible in it. First, the initial and final five seconds of the signal are cropped to remove sections in which voluntary hand movements are expected. After calculating the sample's average framerate, the signal is passed through a 5th order lowpass filter with a cutoff frequency of 20 Hz. This cutoff frequency was chosen taking into consideration that the Parkinsonian tremor frequency range is 3 to 7 Hz, and the hand tremor range (including non-parkinsonian tremor) is 3 to 15 Hz. Once cropped and filtered, we proceeded with feature extraction. We selected features based on the ones described in related publications (*Table 3*), including some new ones, such as the energy in the parkinsonian and hand tremor range.

Features	Description	Calculation
$Avg_{Amplitude}$	Difference between the mean value of the maxima and minima found in $s(t)$. Defining n_{max}, n_{min} as the number of identified maxima and minima. One feature per sample	$\frac{\sum_{i=1}^{n_{max}} \max(s(i))}{n_{max}} - \frac{\sum_{i=1}^{n_{min}} \min(s(i))}{n_{min}}$
Avg_{Signal}	Mean value of $s(t)$, defining n as the length of the sample. One feature per sample	$\frac{\sum_{i=1}^{n} s(i)}{n}$
Std_{Signal}	Standard deviation of $s(t)$. One feature per sample	$\sqrt{\frac{\sum_{i=1}^{n}(s(i) - Avg_{Signal})^2}{n-1}}$
Max_{Signal}, Min_{Signal}	Maximum, minimum of $s(t)$. Two features per sample	$\max(s(t)), \min(s(t))$
$Avg_{Dispersion}$	Average value of the dispersion with a 0.5 second window frame or $\pm n_{Dispersion}$, calculated every 0.05 seconds, resulting in a vector with length $n_{Dispsamples}$. One feature per sample	$Dispersion(t) = \frac{\sum_{i=-n_{Dispersion}}^{n_{Dispersion}} \lvert s(t)-s(i) \rvert}{2\, n_{Dispersion}}$, $Avg_{Dispersion} = \frac{\sum_{i=1}^{n_{Dispsamples}} Dispersion(t)}{n_{Dispsamples}}$
$Std_{Dispersion}$	Standard deviation of the dispersion. One feature per sample	$\sqrt{\frac{\sum_{i=1}^{n}(Dispersion(t) - Avg_{Dispersion})^2}{n_{Dispsamples} - 1}}$
$Energy_{Total}$	Sum of all power spectral densities of the n-point FFT of $s(t)$, defining $PSD(f(i))$ as the spectral energy of $FFT(s)$ at the frequency $f(i) = i(sampling\ rate/n)$	$\sum_{i=1}^{i=n/2} PSD(f(i))$
$Energy_{Tremor}$	Sum of all power spectral densities of the FFT in the tremor range (3 to 15 Hz)	$\sum_{f(i)=3Hz}^{15\ Hz} PSD(f(i))$
$Energy_{PD}$	Sum of all power spectral densities of the FFT in the PD range (3 to 7 Hz)	$\sum_{f(i)=3Hz}^{7\ Hz} PSD(f(i))$
$Energy_{Dominant}$	Power spectral density of the maximum of the FFT	$\max(PSD(f(i))$
$Energy_{Frequency}$	FFT frequency where $Energy_{Dominant}$ was found (usually close to 5 Hz in PD patients)	$f(i) : PSD(f(i)) = Energy_{Dominant}$

Table 21: PALM Task 1 features

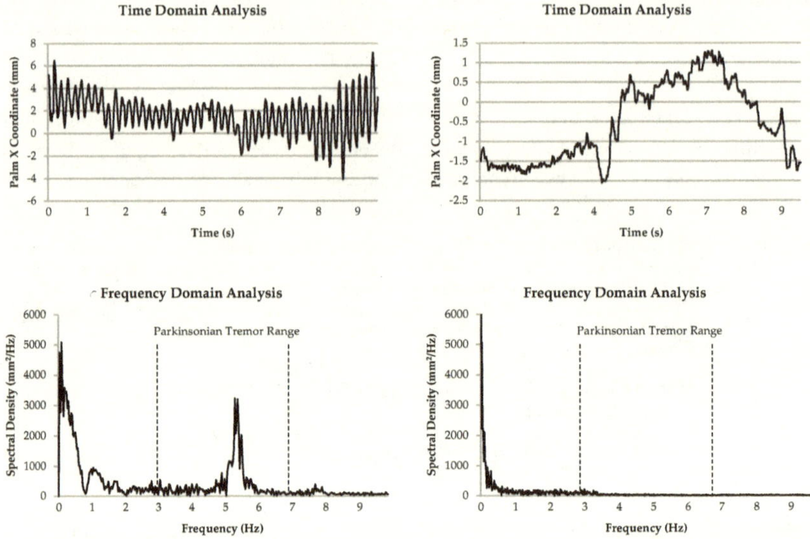

Figure 32: PALM Task 1 sample of a PD patient with severe tremor at OFF (left) and ON (right)

Task 2: Finger Tapping

The goal of Task 2 (*Figure 33*) is to detect speed and amplitude alterations when performing up to ten index and thumb finger taps. In this case, the signal of interest is the difference in the x coordinates of the thumb and index fingers, which should tend to zero when a tap occurs. We chose this signal instead of the provided pinch strength because we found it to have a greater resolution. This signal is normalized by the length of the index finger measured by the Leap Motion sensor, that is:

$$s_1(t) = \frac{tip_{position_{2_x}}(t) - tip_{position_{1_x}}(t)}{\max\left(length_2\right)}$$

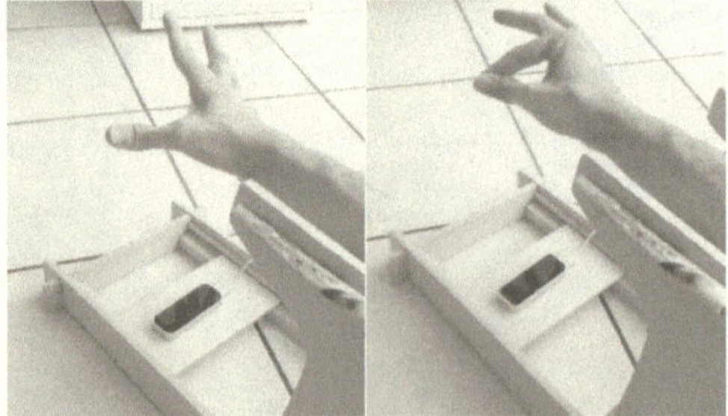

Figure 33: PALM Task 2

The coordinates are described in *Table 19* and the resulting signal (before and after normalization) is depicted in *Figure 34*. The different elements of the kinetic analysis are shown in *Figure 35*. After obtaining the signal, the framerate is calculated and the bandpass filter is applied. The signal is then processed following the steps described in the section *Kinetic Signal Processing*. Afterwards, the features described in *Table 22* are extracted. We chose these features based on the ones described in the related work (*Table 4*), including some that have not yet been tested, such as the duration of open and closed hand periods and polynomial amplitude tendency. After collecting results from several PD patients, we noticed both resting and kinetic tremors are most visible in the palm of the hand. For this reason, all frequency domain features are still collected from the signal:

$$s_2(t) = palm_{position_x}(t)$$

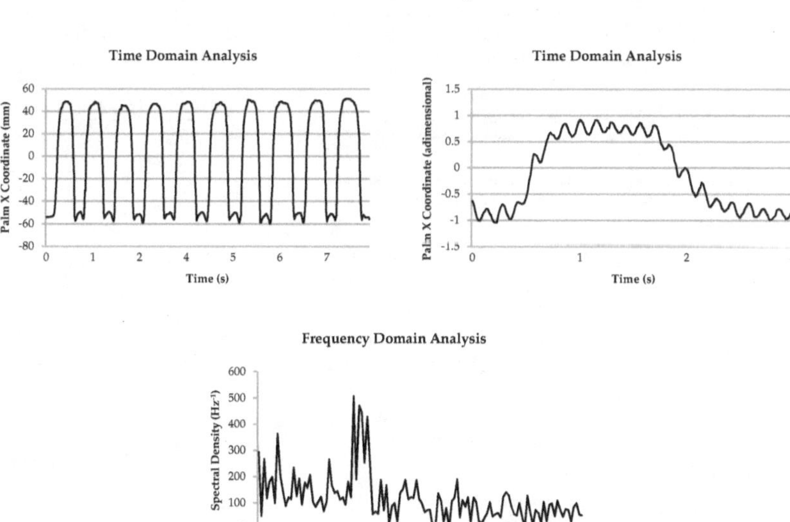

Figure 34: PALM Task 2 sample before normalization (top left), closeup of a repetition with very visible kinetic tremor normalized by finger length (top right), and frequency-domain analysis (bottom)

Features	Description	Calculation
$Time_{Normalized}$	Total time divided by the number of detected repetitions, defined as n_{Rep}. One feature per task	$\frac{Total\ Time}{n_{Rep}}$
Amp_{Mean}	Mean repetition amplitude (see *Kinetic Signal Processing*). One feature per task	$\frac{\sum_{i=1}^{n_{Rep}} Amp(i)}{n_{Rep}}$
Amp_{Std}	Standard deviation of repetition amplitudes. One feature per task	$\sqrt{\frac{\sum_{i=1}^{n_{Rep}} (Amp(i) - Amp_{Mean})^2}{n_{Rep} - 1}}$
Amp_{Max}, Amp_{Min}	Maximum and minimum repetition amplitudes. Two features per task	$\max(Amp(i)), \min(Amp(i))$
$Amp_{Tendency}$	Polynomial coefficient of the least squares first degree polynomial approximation of the signal. One feature per task	Matlab polynomial curve fitting (polyfit)
$Opentime_{Mean}$, $Closedtime_{Mean}$	Mean duration of open and closed hand periods (see *Kinetic Signal Processing*). Two features per task	$\frac{\sum_{i=1}^{n_{Rep}-1} Opentime(i)}{n_{Rep}-1}, \frac{\sum_{i=1}^{n_{Rep}-1} Closedtime(i)}{n_{Rep}-1}$
$Opentime_{Std}$, $Closedtime_{Std}$	Standard deviation of open and closed hand periods. Two features per task	$\sqrt{\frac{\sum_{i=1}^{n_{Rep}-1} (Opentime(i) - Opentime_{Mean})^2}{n_{Rep} - 2}}$
$Speed_{Mean}$	Average speed, including opening and closing speeds (see *Kinetic Signal Processing*). One feature per task	$\frac{\sum_{i=1}^{n_{Rep}-1} Speed(i)}{n_{Rep} - 1}$
$Speed_{Std}$	Standard deviation of speeds, including opening and closing speeds. One feature per task	$\sqrt{\frac{\sum_{i=1}^{n_{Rep}-1} (Speed(i) - Speed_{Mean})^2}{n_{Rep} - 2}}$
$Opening_{Mean}, Opening_{Std}$ $Closing_{Mean}, Closing_{Std}$	Mean and standard deviation of opening and closing speeds. Four features per task	As $Speed_{Mean}$, $Speed_{Std}$ only for $Speed(i) < 0$ (opening) and for $Speed(i) > 0$ (closing)
$Opening_{Max}, Opening_{Min}$	Maximum and minimum of opening speeds. Two features per task	$\max(Speed(i)), \min(Speed(i)), Speed(i) < 0$
$Closing_{Max}, Closing_{Min}$	Maximum and minimum of closing speeds. Two features per task	As $Opening_{Max}$, $Opening_{Min}$, only for $Speed(i) > 0$
$Energy_{Total}$	Sum of all power spectral densities of the n-point FFT of $s_2(t)$, defining $PSD(f(i))$ as the spectral energy of $FFT(s)$ at the frequency $f(i) = i(sampling\ rate/n)$	$\sum_{i=1}^{i=n/2} PSD(f(i))$
$Energy_{Tremor}$	Sum of all power spectral densities of the FFT in the tremor range (3 to 15 Hz).	$\sum_{f(i)=3Hz}^{15\ Hz} PSD(f(i))$
$Energy_{PD}$	Sum of all power spectral densities of the FFT in the PD range (3 to 7 Hz)	$\sum_{f(i)=3Hz}^{7\ Hz} PSD(f(i))$
$Energy_{Dominant}$	Power spectral density of the maximum of the FFT	$\max(PSD(f(i))$
$Energy_{Frequency}$	FFT frequency where $Energy_{Dominant}$ was found (usually close to 5 Hz in PD patients)	$f(i) : PSD(f(i)) = Energy_{Dominant}$

Table 22: PALM Task 2 features

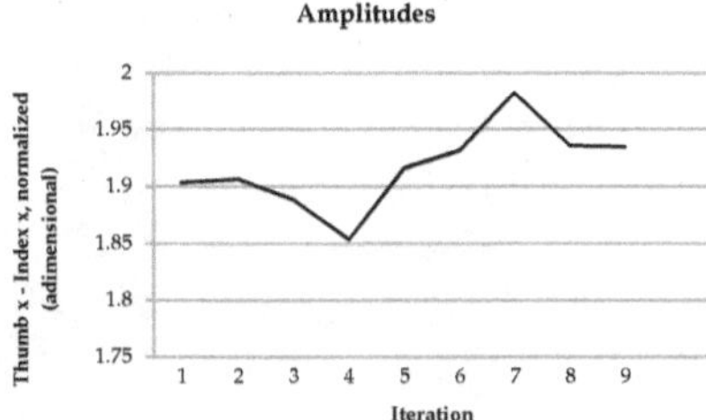

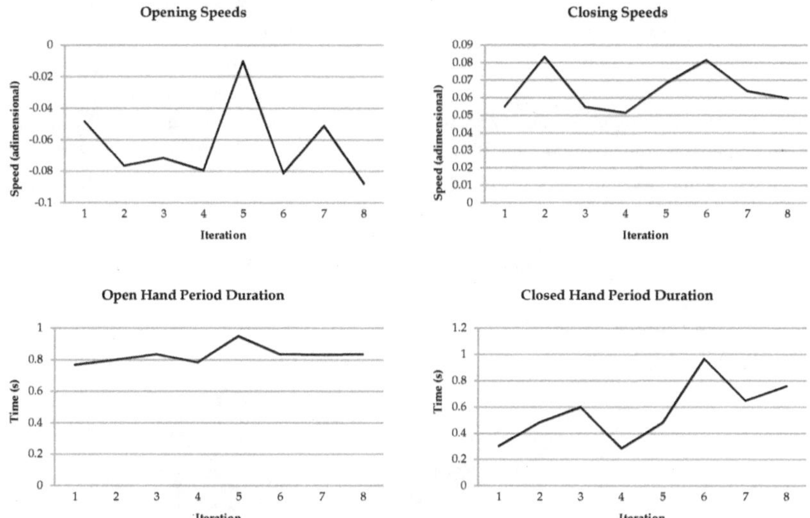

Figure 35: PALM kinetic analysis of a signal from a PD patient

Task 3: Fist Closing

In Task 3 (*Figure 36*), the goal is to detect alterations in a fist opening and closing movement. To study this movement, we calculate the z coordinate of the middle finger minus the z coordinate of the palm center, normalized by finger length. To detect kinetic tremor, we again consider the palm center of the hand, that is:

$$s_1(t) = \frac{tip_{position_{3_z}}(t) - palm_{position_{1_z}}(t)}{\max\,(length_3)},\ s_2(t) = palm_{position_x}(t)$$

We chose this signal instead of the provided grab strength because, as is the case of the previous task, it provided a higher resolution. Signal processing is performed in the same way as Task 2, and the same features, described in *Table 22*, are obtained.

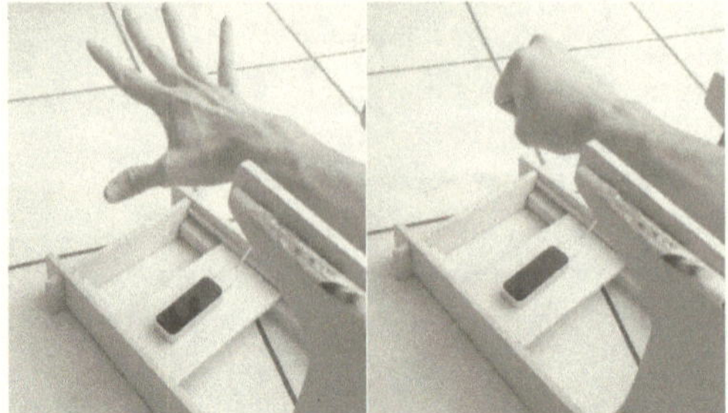

Figure 36: PALM Task 3

Task 4: Pronation-Supination

In the fourth task (*Figure 37*) we analyze a pronation and supination of the hand. The signal to be analyzed is the x coordinate of the thumb, normalized by its length. We also consider kinetic tremor based on the palm of the hand. The extracted features are similar to Task 2 and are thus described in *Table* 22.

$$s_1(t) = \frac{tip_{position_{1_x}}(t)}{\max(length_1)}, s_2(t) = palm_{position_x}(t)$$

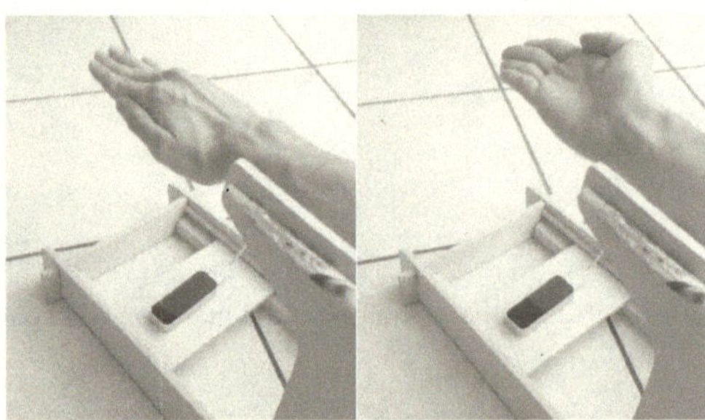

Figure 37: PALM Task 4

Task 5: Lateral Movement

The fifth and last task (*Figure 38*) is not present in the UPDRS test, but is nevertheless of interest to determine hand dexterity and tremors when performing arm movements. In this case, the x coordinate of the palm center is used for analysis. Kinetic tremor may also be present during this task. Signal processing is also similar to Task 2 and thus the features are described in *Table 22*.

$$s(t) = palm_{position_x}(t)$$

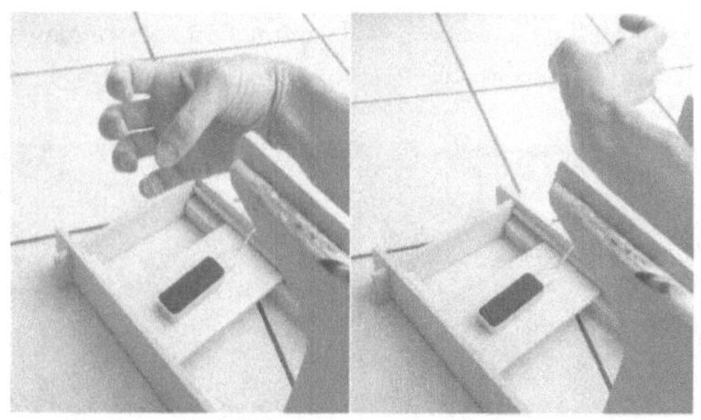

Figure 38: PALM Task 5

6.2. Exergame

Once a data acquisition system was conceived, the next step was to design an exergame to provide an engaging environment for data acquisition. In this case, the requirement was to design an exergame that included a cognitive task and a motor task, controlled with the Leap Motion Sensor. More particularly, the control pattern had to replicate the hand movements performed for the data acquisition of PALM. To achieve this goal, we designed the exergame PDPuzzleTable [93]. This is achieved by implementing a series of puzzles, chosen in collaboration with clinical psychologists for their suitability. The puzzles are controlled with the same hand movements as the ones performed in PALM, so that the same information can be gained. In this sense, the data extracted from PDPuzzleTable can be used to evaluate resting tremor, kinetic tremor, bradykinesia and ON/OFF periods.

In PDPuzzleTable, we present two scenarios. The first scenario is a "Tower of Hanoi" (*Figure 39*). Initially implemented in [65], it is a puzzle consisting of three columns and a set of discs, which are initially in the leftmost column. The goal of the puzzle is to move the discs, one by one, to the rightmost column. It is only possible to place a disk on an empty column, or above a larger disc, limiting the number of possible movements. This task contains two cognitive areas: problem solving and sequencing.

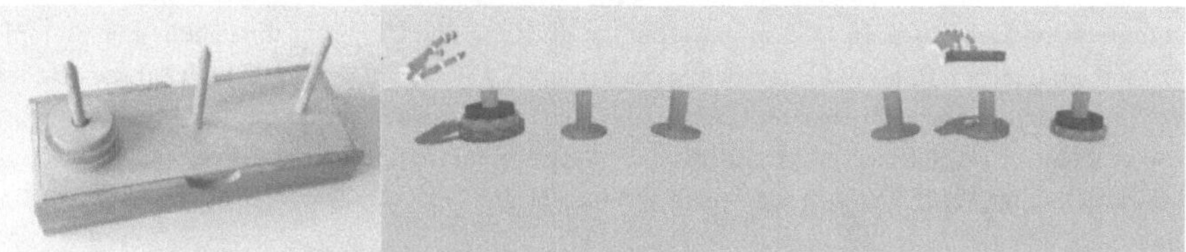

Figure 39: Physical Tower of Hanoi (left) and digital implementation (right) [93]

The second scenario, initially implemented in [302], is a combination of the Corsi block tapping task [158] and the Simon memory game [257]. In this scenario, the player has to observe visual and musical cues emitted by a set of blocks, and repeat the same sequence (*Figure 40*). For every successful cycle, the sequence is extended by one additional element. The game continues until a mistake in the sequence is made. It is also possible to limit the sequence to visual or musical cues, or request the player to complete the sequence backwards. This game addresses the cognitive areas of working memory and sequencing.

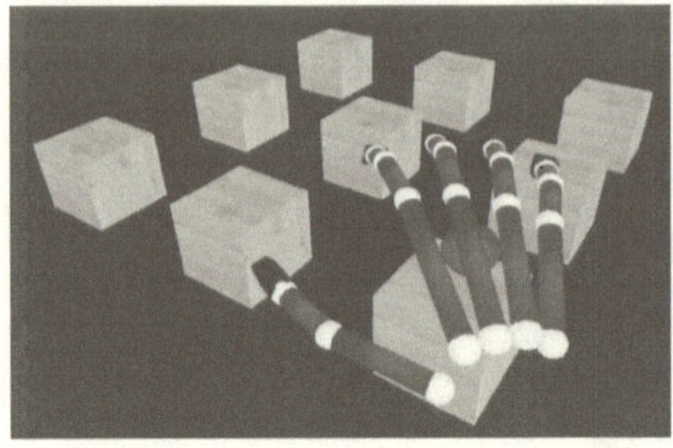 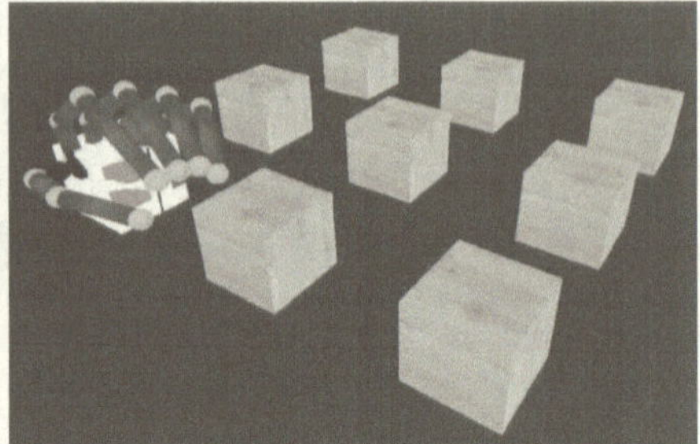

Figure 40: Simon/Corsi memory game digital implementation [302]

In order for the player to interact with the game, we use raw sensor data extracted from LeapC (*Table 19*). In this case, we focus on the parameters *grab_strength* and *pinch_strength* to program interactions, and thus implement two actions: Grabbing, implemented by closing the fist, and pinching, implemented by performing a tap with the index finger and thumb. Although the analysis of hand movements to detect tremor and bradykinesia requires more complex signal analysis, it is sufficient to use these two parameters to program interactions. However, we had to significantly adapt the playability for the limited hand dexterity of PD patients, who in numerous cases have difficulties even with the physical Tower of Hanoi and Simon game, both cognitively and physically.

In order to overcome these difficulties, we introduced visual cues that indicate potential interactions. For example, when hovering the hand over a certain disk in the Tower of Hanoi or a block in the Corsi/Simon game, a blinking object indicates a potential interaction is possible. If the player then performs a pinch or a grab, the interaction occurs.

The actual sensor value that triggers this interaction can be adjusted in both directions. For example, closing the hand to a certain threshold point (e.g., *grab_strength* > 0.8) may count as a grabbing action, and opening the hand again (*grab_strength* < 0.8) drops the object. However, we noticed that tremors make this strategy unfeasible, since the actual value oscillates severely, triggering the threshold continuously. Hence, we decided to decouple the grabbing and dropping thresholds. For example, when the interaction threshold is reached (*grab_strength* > 0.8) an object is grabbed. Afterwards, it is not dropped until a new threshold is reached (*grab_strength* < 0.6). This decoupling greatly removed the problem of involuntary grabs and drops. To further improve this interaction, we included an interaction timer. When an object is dropped, it cannot be grabbed again for a number of seconds (action timer).

Since the interaction in the Tower of Hanoi game is significantly more complex, further adaptations were necessary. First, a visual warning text is presented in case the intended movement is not possible. Second, in some cases, a disc may be dropped mid-air or left in an invalid position. In this case, after a few seconds (reset timer), it can be returned to its latest valid position.

In order to simplify the difficulty adjustment procedure, we implemented preset difficulty levels, as described in *Table 23*. All these mechanics can be toned down or removed completely, which means players would require finer hand control and dexterity to solve the puzzle. In the cognitive domain, the number of elements can be altered (number of discs in the Tower of Hanoi, or number of blocks in the Simon/Corsi game), and the elements can be made to be similar to one another. For example, all blocks in the Simon/Corsi game may have the same texture, or the order can be presented only with visual or auditory cues. In the Tower of Hanoi, all discs can have the same size and only be differentiated by color. These options can be edited for each game session as presented below. In both scenarios, a simple tutorial with a video introduction was created to explain the interaction techniques. This consists of one disc with two towers for the Tower of Hanoi scenario, and two blocks with a two-element sequence for the Simon/Corsi game.

Cognitive difficulty levels	C1	C2	C3	C4	C5
Number of elements	3	4	4	5	5
Element distinction	Yes (visual and auditory cues)	Yes	Yes	Yes	No (auditory cues)
Simon/Corsi order	Forward	Forward	Backward	Forward	Backward
Reset timer	2 s	1 s	Disabled	Disabled	Disabled
Action timer	1.5 s	1 s	Disabled	Disabled	Disabled
Warning texts	Yes	No	No	No	No

Motor difficulty levels	M1	M2	M3	M4	M5
Movement types allowed	Only grabs	Grabs and pinches	Grabs and pinches	Grabs and pinches	Grabs and pinches
Minimum grab/pinch strength	0.8	0.8	0.9	1	1
Drop offset	0.5	0.5	0.25	0.25	0

Table 23: PDPuzzleTable difficulty levels

The features obtained from sensor data are extracted as described in the section *PALM Task Description and Features*, for a window of one second before and after an interaction is recorded. Depending on the interaction options chosen, different signals are taken into consideration. In all cases, the signals are the same as in the respective PALM task. Pinches are processed as described in *Task 2: Finger Tapping*, while grabs are processed as described in *Task 3: Fist Closing*. *Table 24* includes a description of the cognitive feature vector of PDPuzzleTable.

Features	Description	Features	Description
Cognitive difficulty	Cognitive difficulty level of the session (*Table 23*)	Element distinction	Use of same-sized discs (Hanoi) or auditory cues only (Simon) if disabled
Motor difficulty	Motor difficulty level of the session (*Table 23*)	Number of errors	Number of times a non-valid movement was attempted (Hanoi)
Number of actions	Total number of actions until puzzle completion (Hanoi) or failure (Simon)	Movement type	For each action, type of movement (pinch, or grab)
Number of elements	Number of discs (Hanoi) or blocks (Simon) present in game round	Movement origin and destination	For each action, tower of origin of the movement (Hanoi) and tower of destination (Hanoi) or block (Simon)
Simon/Corsi order	Sequency order (forwards or backwards)	Reset timer	Time limit to automatically place back a disc left in the air in its last valid position (Hanoi)
Movement types allowed	Allowed movement types (pinches, grabs, both)	Action timer	Minimum time before an action with an object recently interacted with is allowed again
Minimum grab/pinch strength	Interaction threshold values for grabbing (Hanoi and Simon)	Total time	Total game Time
Drop offset	Offset value for dropping threshold (Hanoi)	Time per movement	Time elapsed between each movement

Table 24: PDPuzzleTable game data features

6.3. Evaluation

Cohort and Study Design

The evaluation of this clinical decision support system should determine its accuracy in assessing whether the player has parkinsonian tremor and bradykinesia. Initially, we had planned an evaluation, to commence in March 2019, using PDPuzzleTable to classify PD patients and healthy controls and predict the UPDRS scores of Tasks 3.4 to 3.6, 3.15, and 3.16. This evaluation was firstly delayed due to modifications required by the ethics committee prior to approval. After we finally obtained approval in March 2020, it was again delayed due to the COVID-19 pandemic. Instead, we present an evaluation based on the preliminary data we collected to design PALM, particularly its signal processing and choice of classification features.

For this evaluation, we use a diagnosis of PD as our clinical outcome. Each participant performs all five tasks of PALM with both hands. This means that for each task, we obtain two samples per participant. The goal of our system is to classify whether the participant has PD or is a healthy control. The system diagram, as conceived in *Chapter 4*, is depicted in *Figure 41*. For this evaluation we use the features described in the section *PALM Task Description and Features*, *Table 21* and *Table 22*.

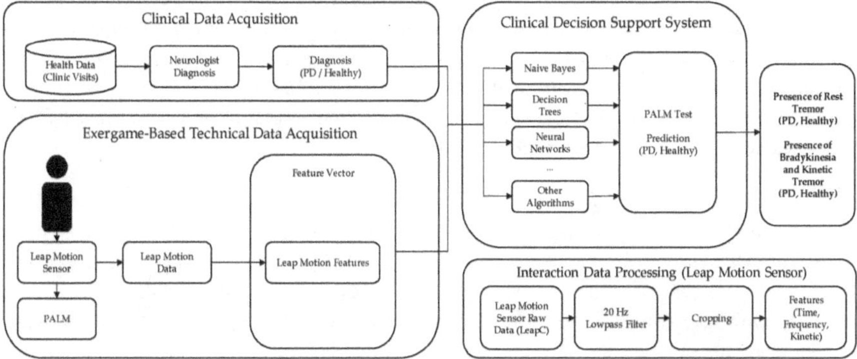

Figure 41: Exergame-based clinical decision support system to assess hand tremor and bradykinesia. System diagram

For this evaluation, a cohort of 10 participants (*Table 52*, median age 59, three males) were selected and recruited at the Schmieder neurology clinics in Konstanz and Allensbach, as well as at the Westrich Ergotherapeutic practice in Mannheim. Information about PD participants is provided in *Appendix F, Table 59*. Control participants were recruited at the Multimedia Communications Lab of the Technical University of Darmstadt. For the PD group, the inclusion criterion was an age of 50 or older and the positive diagnosis of PD by a neurologist, and the exclusion criterion was the presence of coexisting neurological or otherwise chronic diseases affecting hand dexterity. For the control group, the inclusion criterion was an age of 50 or older, and the exclusion criteria were the presence of any neurological disease or diseases causing hand tremors. Each participant performed all PALM tasks with the right and left hands. In order to increase the sample size, each hand was considered as a separate sample. This means we had a total of 20 samples per task for classification. All participants signed an informed consent prior to participation, presented in *Appendix F*.

We consider two separate evaluation scenarios. In the first scenario, we attempt to discriminate PD patients and controls based on PALM Task 1. This task is designed to detect PD resting tremor. In the second scenario, we attempt to discriminate PD patients and controls based on PALM Tasks 2 to 5. These tasks discriminate based on bradykinesia and kinetic tremor. The tasks use the same features, collected for different exercises. One PD patient had a very significant hand tremor and was unable to perform these tasks. We present the classification results for a combination of all tasks. Effect sizes for the first scenario are described in *Appendix F, Table 60*, while the effect sizes for the second scenario are included in *Table 65* and *Table 66*.

Results for Resting Tremor

As shown in *Table 26* and *Figure 42*, PALM can accurately discriminate PD patients from healthy controls in our cohort. Both algorithms misclassified the same sample, belonging to PD patient P02. As described in *Appendix F, Table 59*, P02 is a patient with a very recent diagnosis of PD, who was under the effect of medication when the sample was taken. When analyzing all samples of P02 visually, we unfortunately did not identify any possible features or other differences that may be used for classification. Concerning effect sizes, as presented in *Table 60,* no features showed statistical significance. However, we believe this is due to the small sample size. Algorithm hyperparameters are described in *Appendix D, Table 50.* In order to make sure that data leakage did not influence our results (training the algorithm with the left hand of a PD patient and testing on the right), we tested the algorithms using only one sample per patient. Classification results were similar considering the sample size was halved to 10 vectors (90% accuracy).

Results for Kinetic Tremor and Bradykinesia

In *Table 27* and *Figure 43,* we provide the classification results using the features of all tasks combined. Task-specific classification results are provided in *Appendix F, Table 61* to *Table 64* and *Figure 64* to *Figure 67.* All samples except one from P02 were again correctly classified. When considering the tasks separately, we achieved 100% accuracy in Task 2 (*Table 61*) and Task 5 (*Table 64*), although this was not unlikely given the sample size. Algorithm accuracy varied greatly between tasks. For example, we achieved this accuracy in Task 5 using a neural network, but this same algorithm resulted in a performance of 72% in Task 3. As was the case in the previous scenario, we could not visually or analytically see differences between P02 and the control group. Concerning effect sizes, we identified statistically significant features with large effect sizes in all the tasks (*Table 65, Table 66).* The features that were consistently identified as statistically significant are described in *Table 25.* Again, data leakage does not seem to have an impact in our cohort.

Feature	Significant ($p<0.05$) in PALM tasks	Effect Size (g)
$Time_{Normalized}$	5	1.6248
Amp_{Mean}	2	-1.6706
Amp_{Std}	2	-1.6621
Amp_{Max}	2,5	-1.4477, -1.5759
$Speed_{Mean}$	2,4,5	-2.0639, -1.4749, -2.2489
$Speed_{Std}$	2,4	-2.2738, -1.5617
$Opening_{Mean}$	All	1.6005, 1.5845, 1.5627, 2.4206
$Opening_{Std}$	4,5	-1.2481, -1.4205
$Opening_{Max}$	5	2.1207
$Opening_{Min}$	All	1.8057, 1.64, 1.6754, 2.5346
$Closing_{Mean}$	2,4	-2.1894, -1.3671
$Closing_{Std}$	5	-1.622
$Closing_{Max}$	2,4	-1.7979, -1.5815
$Closing_{Min}$	2,5	-1.8707, -2.0636

Table 25: PALM Tasks 2 to 5 classification results. Effect sizes of statistically significant features in different tasks

Algorithm: Naïve Bayes, accuracy 95.000%	Correctly classified	Incorrectly classified	TP rate	FP rate	Precision	F	MCC	ROC area	PRC area
PD	9 (TP)	1 (FN)	0.900	0	1	0.947	0.905	0.900	0.950
Control	10 (TN)	0 (FP)	1	0.100	0.909	0.952	0.905	0.900	0.798
Weighted average	19	1	0.950	0.050	0.955	0.950	0.905	0.900	0.874
Algorithm: Hoeffding Tree, accuracy 95.000%									
PD	9 (TP)	1 (FN)	0.900	0	1	0.947	0.905	0.900	0.950
Control	10 (TN)	0 (FP)	1	0.100	0.909	0.952	0.905	0.900	0.798
Weighted average	19	1	0.950	0.050	0.955	0.950	0.905	0.900	0.874

Table 26: PALM Task 1 classification results

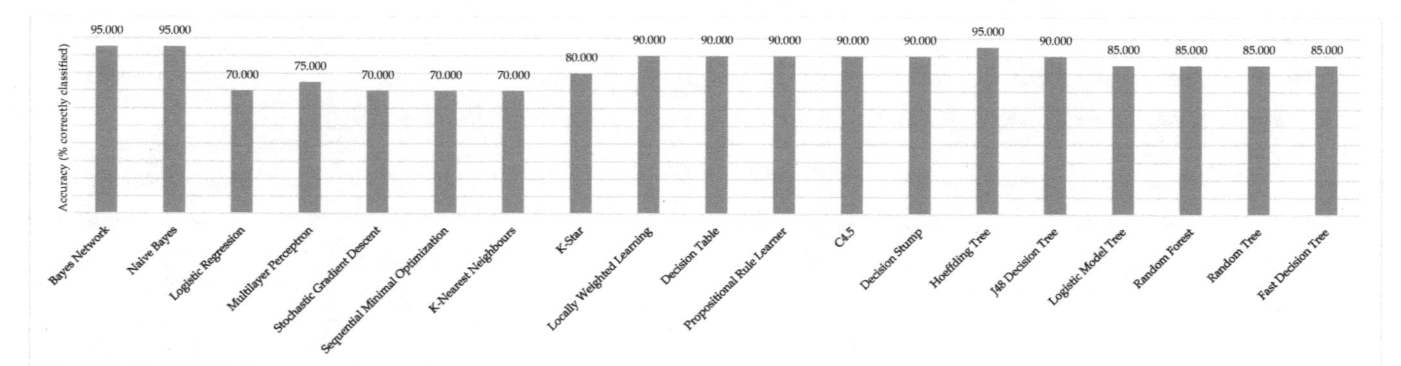

Figure 42: PALM Task 1 classification accuracies

Algorithm: Naïve Bayes, accuracy 94.44%	Correctly classified	Incorrectly classified	TP rate	FP rate	Precision	F	MCC	ROC area	PRC area
PD	7 (TP)	1 (FN)	0.875	0	1	0.933	0.892	0.988	0.986
Control	10 (TN)	0 (FP)	1	0.125	0.909	0.952	0.892	0.938	0.909
Weighted average	17	1	0.944	0.069	0.949	0.944	0.892	0.960	0.943
Algorithm: Hoeffding Tree, accuracy 94.44%									
PD	7	1	0.875	0	1	0.933	0.892	0.975	0.975
Control	10	0	1	0.125	0.909	0.952	0.892	0.938	0.909
Weighted average	17	1	0.944	0.069	0.949	0.944	0.892	0.954	0.938

Table 27: PALM Tasks 2 to 5 combined classification results

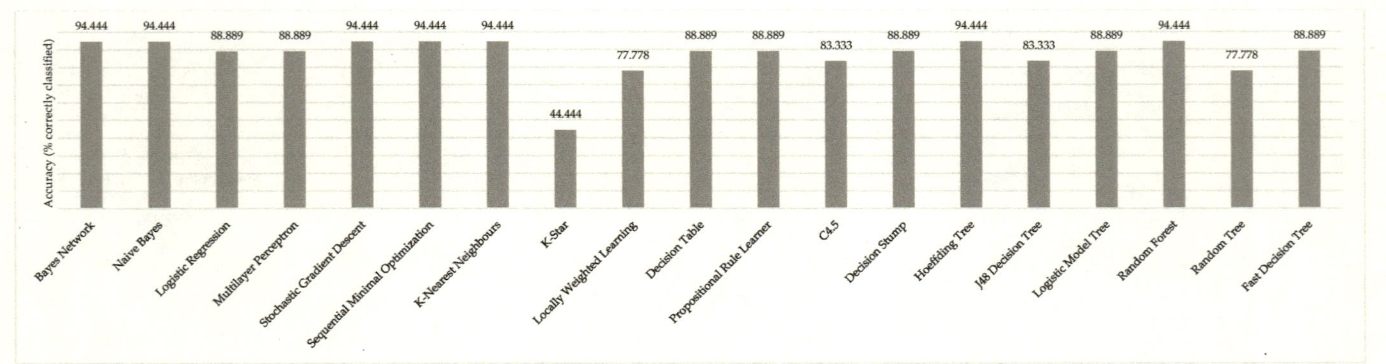

Figure 43: PALM Tasks 2 to 5 combined classification accuracies

PDPuzzleTable Acceptance

The acceptance of PDPuzzleTable was tested with healthy participants. For this acceptance test, 40 participants were invited to play PDPuzzleTable and give their opinion on the game. Before playing, the different input methods and the game concept were presented. Each player played a total of six sessions. In two of these sessions, players used a mouse to play the games, in the remaining four they used the Leap Motion sensor. From these four sessions, two were played by using the lowest difficulty level (C1 and M1, see *Table 23*), and two playing at medium difficulty (C3 and M3). After playing the game, participants were presented with a questionnaire, similar to the one presented in *Appendix E*, section *Extended Balance Board Evaluation. Questionnaires.* Results of this questionnaire are presented in *Figure 44* and *Figure 45*.

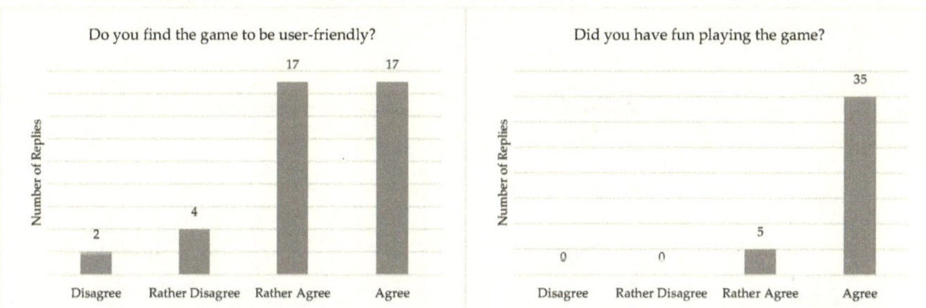

Figure 44: PDPuzzleTable acceptance test results for user-friendliness and fun

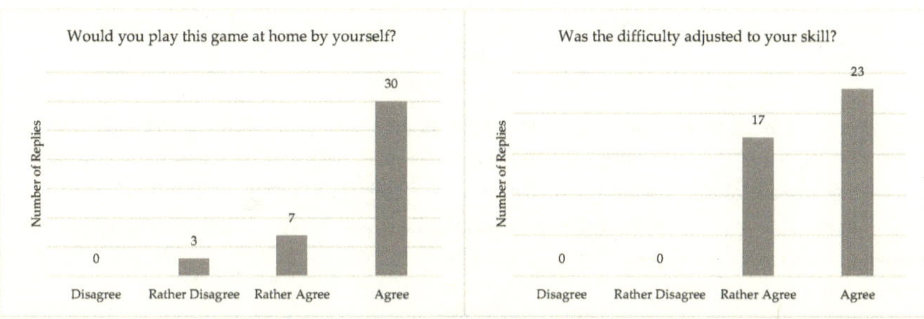

Figure 45: PDPuzzleTable acceptance test results for home monitoring potential and skill adjustment

Regarding usability and control, almost all users found the game to be user-friendly. Most users preferred the Leap Motion sensor over the mouse. After increasing difficulty, we noticed almost all users had at least one involuntary object interaction. In regards to the settings (adjusting the grabbing and pinching threshold to adapt to the player's hand dexterity), all users indicated that the settings did adjust the game to their dexterity.

In addition to this questionnaire, considering that the interaction with the Leap Motion sensor is not as intuitive as the Extended Balance Board, a performance test was made. In this test, we compared the number of movements performed when interacting with the Leap Motion sensor and two traditional methods: mouse interaction for the Simon/Corsi game, and a physical Tower of Hanoi.

As we expected, performance was slightly affected when using the sensor (*Figure 46*). In the case of the Simon/Corsi game, the effect of the sensor in determining cognitive performance is relatively unaffected by difficulty, since the sequence length remained largely unaltered. This was also the case for the Tower of Hanoi game, as long as the difficulty was low. Removing the mechanisms that simplified interaction with the Leap Motion sensor (action and reset timers, minimum grab strength and drop offset) introduced a great number of involuntary interactions, resulting in a significantly higher number of total movements. For this reason, when using PDPuzzleTable to assess cognition, at least with the Tower of Hanoi, it is important to consider that a learning effect can be expected with each difficulty increase, particularly in the difficulty levels when these ease of use mechanisms are disabled (C2 to C3 and M4 to M5).

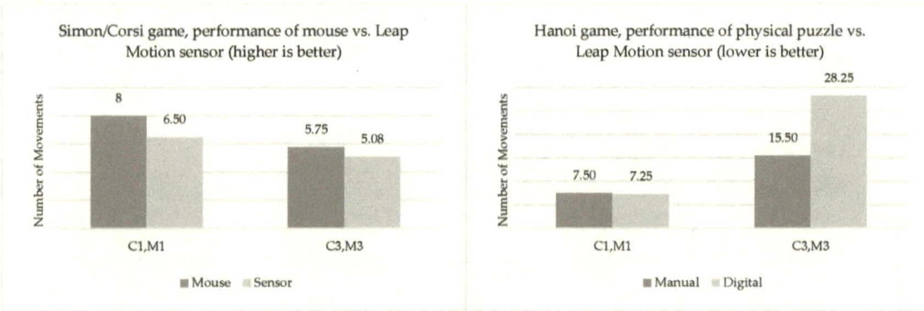

Figure 46: Performance differences when using the Leap Motion sensor vs. mouse and physical puzzle

In summary, the acceptance results of PDPuzzleTable are quite positive in all fields. However, it is important to take the learning effect into consideration: interacting with the Leap Motion sensor is less intuitive than we initially expected. The lower difficulty settings of PDPuzzleTable help to mitigate this effect. A discussion on potential future work based on the results of the evaluation and user acceptance is presented in *Chapter 9*.

7. Additional Biosignal Modules

Chapter 5 and *Chapter 6* present two proofs of concept of exergame-based clinical decision support systems designed to monitor symptoms of PD presented in *Chapter 4*. As described in the system diagram in *Figure 4*, the system uses three data sources: data extracted from the game (game data), from the sensor used to operate the exergame (interaction data) and from the players themselves (biosignals). In this sense, game data can be used to estimate both cognitive and physical symptoms, while interaction data are mostly used to monitor a physical symptom affecting the way the exergame interaction occurs. As a secondary goal of this book, we explored how biosignals may be collected, ideally in the background, to either monitor further symptoms of PD or to provide additional data on an already monitored symptom, thus aiming to increase system accuracy. In *Chapter 3*, section *Sensor-based Approaches to Monitor Symptoms of Parkinson's Disease*, we discussed two such symptoms. These are (1) depressed sympathetic and parasympathetic activity, which can be detected via PPG, and (2) the effect dyskinesia and ON-OFF periods have on the blink-rate. In this chapter, we present algorithms to monitor these two symptoms. First, we present a smartphone-based PPG algorithm that can accurately time heartbeats. We compared our system with the golden clinical standard, ECG. We published this algorithm in [90]. Second, we designed a blink-rate detection algorithm based on a time series that estimates the dimensions of the open eye. We published this algorithm in [94]. This algorithm was tested with two publicly available datasets as well as our own evaluation dataset. Further details are provided in *Appendix G*.

7.1. Heart-rate Estimation Algorithm

As discussed in the section *Depressed Sympathetic and Parasympathetic Cardiac Activity* of *Chapter 3*, sympathetic and parasympathetic dysfunctions are common symptoms of PD. These symptoms can be monitored measuring heart-rate variability, which can be done with PPG [281]. For this purpose, smartphones offer a viable [87, 115, 116, 140] and ubiquitous [233, 249] option. When the user places their finger over the camera lens, a PPG algorithm can detect the exact time when a heartbeat occurs, and then measure the time interval between these heartbeats. In ECG, this interval is called R-R, since it is measured as the amount of time between the two R points of the so-called QRS complex. The PPG signal calculates an approximation of this interval. R-R intervals from healthy heartbeats are commonly referred to as N-N intervals, thus also measuring the amount of time between the two R peaks. Since a PPG algorithm cannot detect these abnormal heartbeats, we also refer to N-N intervals in PPG (*Figure 47*) [332].

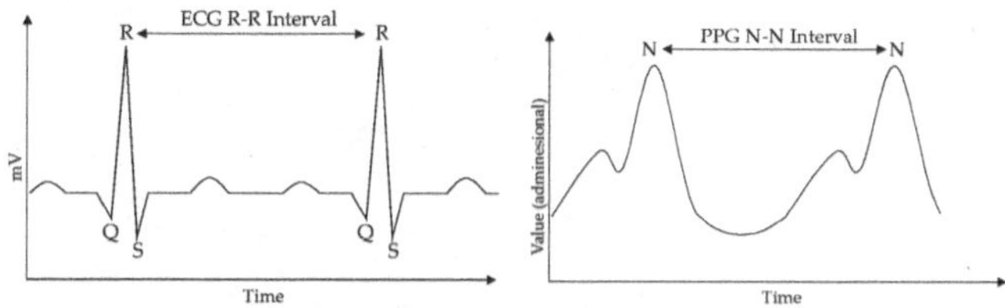

Figure 47: Sketch of a R-R interval measured in the shape of an ECG wave (left) and its approximation in PPG waves (right)

In this book, as part of our secondary goals, we developed a novel PPG algorithm. We included the processing techniques that had provided the best results so far: using the second order difference of the PPG signal [66], bandpass filtering, considering all red, green and blue (RGB) channels [326], and using cubic spline interpolation [6]. We designed a PPG heartbeat detection algorithm that does not require manually editing the signal, and we evaluated its capability to time heartbeats against the gold standard: two-lead ECG.

We produced our PPG signal using a Google LG Nexus 5 capturing videos at a resolution of 1280x960 pixels and a frequency of 30 Hz. This was the highest resolution where real-time signal processing, as described below, was still possible for this smartphone. Using Android Studio [112], we developed an application that captures the video, extracts the frames, and calculates the PPG signal, sending this signal to a computer running Matlab via a wireless ad-hoc network. In practice, we found the actual framerate of the camera to oscillate between 28 and 29 Hz, and the network latency to be 2.76 ms on average. We calculate our photoplethysmographic signal, $ppg(t)$, as follows: for each sampling time t, we have a 1280x960 array of three-pixel values: red, green, and blue. If we define $\mathbf{R}, \mathbf{G}, \mathbf{B} \in \mathbb{R}^{1280\times960}$ as the three matrices representing these RGB values, where $r_{i,j}, g_{i,j}, b_{i,j} \in [0,255]$ represent the RGB values of pixel $(i,)$, we calculate our PPG signal as:

$$ppg(t) = \frac{\sum_{i=1}^{1280}\sum_{j=1}^{960}(r_{i,j} + g_{i,j} + b_{i,j})}{1280 \cdot 960}$$

As a blood pulse circulates through the finger, an oscillatory signal in the three RGB channels is observed. *Figure 48* presents three grayscale frames, as captured directly by the smartphone camera, and a sample of the generated wave $ppg(t)$. We present these frames in grayscale, since it is visually challenging to appreciate this difference in the original frames, which are red in color.

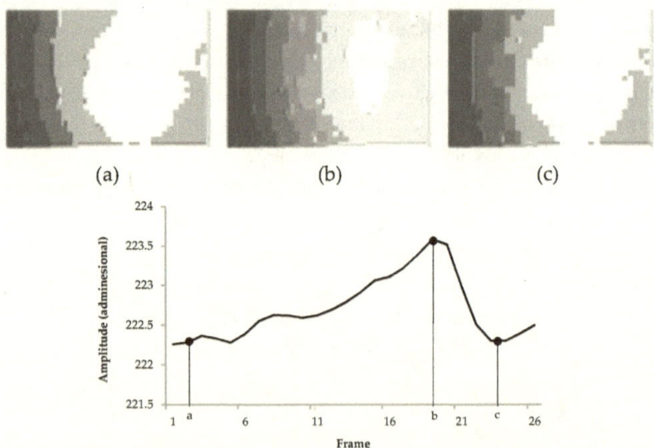

Figure 48: PPG frames captured by a smartphone (top), where a color change due to blood vessel dilation (a vs. b) is visible, and the resulting raw PPG signal (bottom). The points on the signal where the frames were captured are also marked as "a" "b" and "c" [90]

In this PPG signal, it is possible to detect heartbeats using peak detection. We noticed that minima (points a and c in *Figure 48*) were slightly more reliable than maxima (point b in *Figure 48*) due to the shape of the signal. This is because several local maxima in the PPG wave might be falsely identified as heartbeats. However, since the goal is to time heartbeats, both options are possible as long as only one peak is found per oscillation (that is, per heartbeat). We found that a minimum can be determined to be a heartbeat if it is lower than or equal to the surrounding eight frames to the left and right (referring to a 30 Hz signal). This means points a and c in *Figure 48* would be classified as heartbeats, and the time between points a and c would be the $i - th$ N-N interval of a series, or mathematically:

$$nn_{PPG_i} = (c - a) \leftrightarrow \forall x \in [a - 8, a + 8], ppg(a) \leq ppg(x), \forall x \in [c - 8, c + 8], ppg(c) \leq ppg(x)$$

We thus define $\boldsymbol{nn}_{PPG}$ as a vector of N-N intervals in a sample. For a PPG signal to produce a peak in less than 8 frames, the user's heart-rate would have to be over 230 beats per minute, which we do not expect to happen [124]. Also, one could widen this comparison range to reduce the number of potential errors, but that would imply that high heart-rates may not be correctly detected. Although this works well in ideal conditions, even a small body movement or change in ambient light conditions introduces errors in the signal. Under these circumstances, it is necessary to filter the signal. A sample of a signal with artifacts is presented in *Figure 49*.

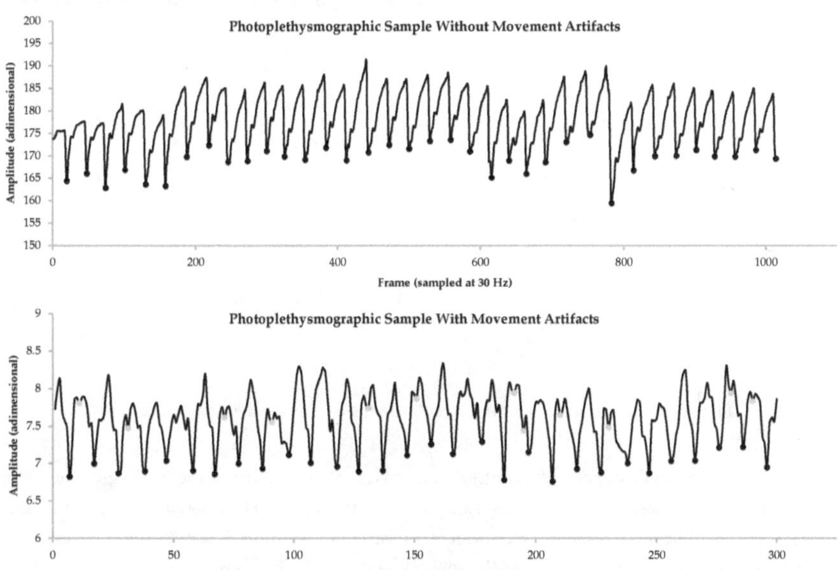

Figure 49: Sample PPG signals without and with movement artifacts. Detected minima are marked as dots, the black dots represent actual heartbeats detected by the algorithm, and the gray dots represent falsely detected heartbeats [90]

After evaluating several filters, we found that employing a 5th order 0.075–2 Hz bandpass filter removed most movement artifacts from the resting users' PPG signals. After filtering, we calculated the second order difference, as suggested in [66]. In the resulting sine wave, heartbeats can be detected by studying complete oscillations based on zero crossings: an increasing zero-crossing, followed by a decreasing zero-crossing counts as a heartbeat. Finally, we noticed two artifacts remained: venous pulsations detected as heartbeats (a local maximum directly before the peak of the PPG wave) and heartbeat skipping (two heartbeats considered to be one). Although these could not be filtered, they can be eliminated. These errors mean a certain heartbeat interval suddenly shows roughly half or double the value of the surrounding heartbeats, which is very unlikely from a physiological perspective. A direct correction method was employed for this problem: heartbeat intervals longer than 1.7 times the surrounding values are halved, and two subsequent intervals, each 0.6 times or less the surrounding values, are merged. We found these two values removed most of these errors without introducing any additional alteration to the signal.

In order to provide our standard comparison, we captured ECG signals in parallel using the g.Tec USBAmp biosignal amplifier, employing active electrodes and a 50 Hz notch filter, with a frequency of 200 Hz. The position of the electrodes is depicted in *Figure 50*. The electrocardiographic signal showed no artifacts, and did not require any further filtering. A simple peak detection algorithm was used to detect the R points as depicted in *Figure 47* and measure the R-R intervals. We visually verified that all R-R intervals were detected correctly. We refer to these intervals as $\boldsymbol{rr}_{ECG}$, a vector of R-R intervals in a given sample.

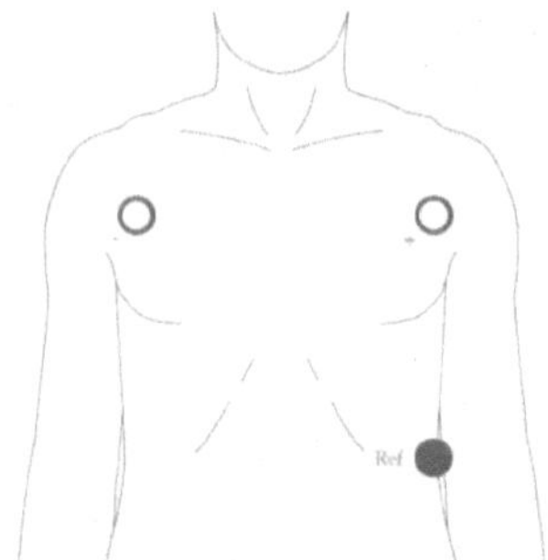

Figure 50: Electrode placement to acquire the ECG signal. Courtesy of [195]

Considering that the PPG signal was captured at approximately 30 Hz and the ECG signal at 200 Hz, the PPG signal was interpolated to the sampling points of the ECG signal using cubic spline interpolation. In addition to network latency, it is important to consider that PPG and ECG heartbeats do not occur physically at the same time. The time required for the blood pulse wave to move from the heart (ECG R point) to the fingertip (PPG N point) has to be considered [148]. In order to solve this, the Pearson correlation was calculated between the ECG and PPG signals while displacing the PPG signal backwards, until maximum correlation was achieved (that is, where R and N points concur the most, final correlation values are provided in *Table 67* and *Table 68*). A diagram of the system is presented in *Figure 51*. In order to compare between ECG R-R and PPG N-N intervals, we used several statistical criteria, as described in *Table 28*.

Feature	Description	Calculation
Err_{Avg}	Average absolute error between PPG and ECG, for a sample with m intervals. Ideally this value would be zero	$\frac{\sum_{i=1}^{m}\lvert nn_{PPG_i} - rr_{ECG_i}\rvert}{m}$
Err_{Std}	Average absolute error of the standard deviation between PPG and ECG, for a sample with n intervals, if we define $\overline{\boldsymbol{nn}}_{PPG}$ and $\overline{\boldsymbol{rr}}_{ECG}$ as the average of PPG and ECG intervals. Ideally this value would be zero	$\sqrt{\frac{\sum_{i=1}^{m}(nn_{PPG_i} - \overline{nn}_{PPG})^2}{m-1}} - \sqrt{\frac{\sum_{i=1}^{m}(rr_{ECG_i} - \overline{rr}_{ECG})^2}{m-1}}$
$Corr$	Pearson correlation coefficient between PPG and ECG. Ideally one	$\frac{\sum_{i=1}^{m}(nn_{PPG_i} - \overline{nn}_{PPG}) \cdot (rr_{ECG_i} - \overline{rr}_{ECG})}{\sqrt{\sum_{i=1}^{m}(nn_{PPG_i} - \overline{nn}_{PPG})^2} \cdot \sqrt{\sum_{i=1}^{m}(rr_{ECG_i} - \overline{rr}_{ECG})^2}}$

Table 28: Heart-rate estimation algorithm features

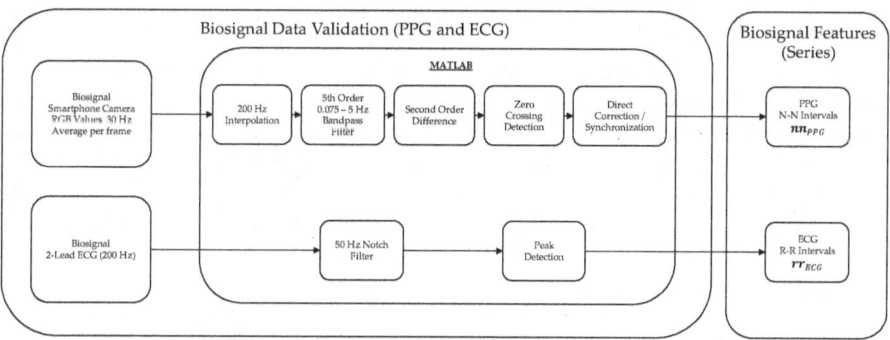

Figure 51: Photoplethysmographic biosignal processing diagram

Evaluation

As the first part of our evaluation, we explored how different resolutions affect the performance and accuracy of the PPG algorithm. For this purpose, we captured 5-minute ECG and PPG signals in parallel using different framerates and resolutions in one user and measured the Err_{Avg}. The results of this analysis are presented in *Figure 52*. We found that increasing resolution does not necessarily improve accuracy, but increasing framerate does, since the performance at 30 Hz is consistently better than at 15 Hz for all resolutions. For the final implementation of our algorithm, we reduced the resolution to 800x600 at 30 Hz to reduce the risk of CPU thermal throttling.

Once we had implemented a final version of our algorithm, we tested it with a cohort of 31 participants. We recruited our participants through university classes. Inclusion criteria were willingness to perform ECG electrode acquisition, while exclusion criteria were the presence of cardiopathies. We recorded ECG and PPG signals in parallel for five minutes while sitting. Sample length was chosen in accordance with the heart-rate variability assessment standards [308]. Users were instructed to hold the smartphone in their hand and gently press the index finger against the camera lens. They were encouraged to change their sitting position to introduce movement artifacts.

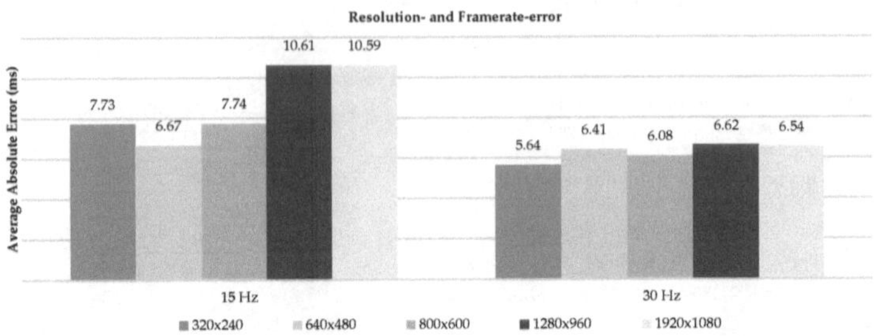

Figure 52: Absolute error of the PPG algorithm when using different resolutions and framerates [90]

We evaluated three different PPG algorithms: an unfiltered minima detection algorithm (*Figure 49)*, a filtered minima detection algorithm, and the complete algorithm including second degree differentiation, zero-crossing detection and direct correction. In all cases, the correlation-based synchronization procedure was performed. The average results are presented in *Table 29*, and complete per-user results are available in *Appendix G, Table 67* and *Table 68*. In addition, we present graphical examples of four characteristic users: 2 for its low Err_{Avg}, 5 for its low $Corr$, 18 for its high $Corr$ and 25 for its high Err_{Avg}, in *Figure 53*. The Bland-Altman plots of these same users, depicting the error in each interval, are presented in *Figure 54*.

Algorithm	Err_{Avg} (ms)	Err_{Std} (ms)	$Corr$ (adimensional)
Unfiltered algorithm	28.58	58.75	0.29
Filtered algorithm	11.12	84.49	0.68
Novel algorithm	9.23	85.32	0.65

Table 29: PPG algorithm average results for all users

These results display the excellent performance of the developed algorithm, which shows an average absolute error of 9.23 ms, much lower than the other approaches. However, performance shows significant interindividual differences: the system performed quite poorly in some users, for example user 25 (see *Figure 53*). Given that the unfiltered approach does not show this error, further optimizing the filter parameters may solve this issue. However, the raw data do not show any significant differences in comparison with other users that would elicit this decrease in performance. Correlation ($Corr = 0.65$) and standard deviation ($Err_{Std} = 85.32$) results are less ideal. However, this does not seem to impact the main results: despite of the disparity of $Corr$ values in users 5 and 18, the algorithm seems to accurately track heartbeats in both users. Perhaps a more sophisticated filtering method would improve these results. Another potential improvement point is the artifact removal procedure. On the example of user 2, the algorithm still miscalculates some intervals due to these artifacts, even in the users where it provided the best performance.

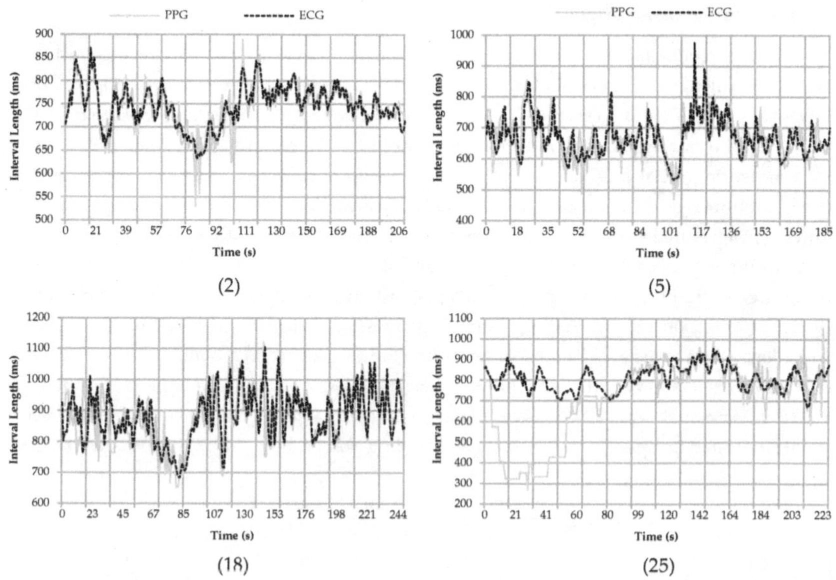

Figure 53: PPG evaluation, absolute error graphical results. User number indicated below the image

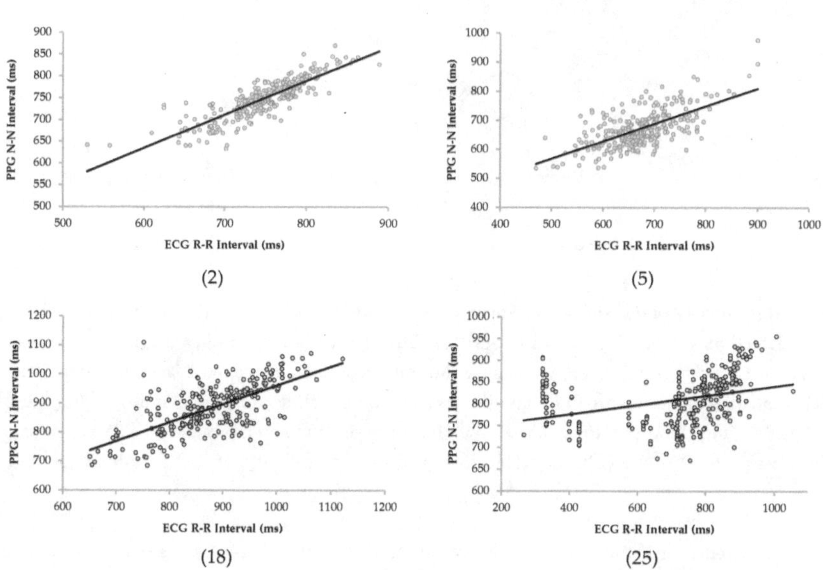

Figure 54: PPG evaluation, Bland-Altman graphical results. User number indicated below the image

7.2. Blink-rate Estimation Algorithm

As discussed in the section *Blink-rate* of *Chapter 3*, one of the multiple ways bradykinesia manifests itself in PD is with a reduction of the eye blink-rate [22, 150, 309]. This reduction seems to disappear during ON periods [163, 309]. This suggests that blink-rate monitoring could be potentially used to track ON-OFF periods non-invasively and determine the severity of bradykinesia. As an alternative to detecting eye blinks measuring facial muscular activity, which would require electrodes, we implemented a method based on images captured by a webcam [234]. Instead of implementing a classifier to detect blinks directly, we wanted to provide a time series that would be representative of eye activity. Once validated, this time series could be used to provide additional information on blinks, such as opening and closing speeds. In this sense, we developed an algorithm that extends the work of Soukupová et al. [290] and is based on the Eye Aspect Ratio (EAR). $EAR(t)$ is calculated based on the distances between six key points of the eye (*Figure 55*). According to [290], $EAR(t)$ is around 0.25 when the eye is open, and rapidly tends to zero during a blink. When the EAR is below 0.2, a blink is considered to have occurred. Mathematically, $EAR(t)$ is calculated as follows: let $\boldsymbol{p_1}(t)$ to $\boldsymbol{p_6}(t)$ be coordinate vectors of the points indicated in *Figure 55* in the frame of sampling point t, then $EAR(t)$ is calculated as [290]:

$$EAR(t) = \frac{\|\boldsymbol{p_2}(t) - \boldsymbol{p_6}(t)\| + \|\boldsymbol{p_3}(t) - \boldsymbol{p_5}(t)\|}{2\|\boldsymbol{p_1}(t) - \boldsymbol{p_4}(t)\|}$$

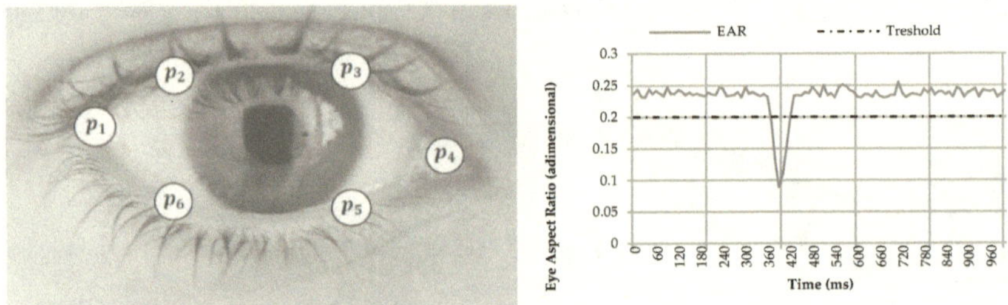

Figure 55: Eye aspect ratio calculation points and resulting function

The algorithm consists of five steps: (1) frame acquisition and preprocessing, (2) face detection, (3) facial features detection, (4) pupil positioning and (5) $EAR(t)$ calculation. Frames are first converted to grayscale and preprocessed. Then, we ensure the frame contains a face, and facial features. Finally, $EAR(t)$ is calculated. Frames are then classified as containing a blink or not, depending on the value of $EAR(t)$ at that frame and previous values. The algorithm depends on a number of external functions and libraries from OpenCV [239] and Dlib [59]. The five components of the algorithm function as follows:

For each captured frame, the frame acquisition module (1) retrieves a $i \times j \times 3$ matrix, in our case $640 \times 480 \times 3$, where 640×480 is the camera resolution, and 3 represents the three RGB channels. The image is converted to grayscale and reduced in size by a factor of four to speed up the process. This is done as follows: let $\mathbf{R}, \mathbf{G}, \mathbf{B} \in \mathbb{R}^{640\times480}$ be the gamma-normalized matrix of RGB values for a given image, then we define a new matrix, intensity $\mathbf{I}_l$ as:

$$\mathbf{I}_i = \frac{1}{3}(\mathbf{R} + \mathbf{G} + \mathbf{B})$$

We then reduce the size of $\mathbf{I}_i$ to $\mathbf{I} \in \mathbb{R}^{320\times240}$ by calculating the average of each four-element block. Using this matrix **I**, we perform facial detection (2) as implemented by Dalal and Triggs [51]. First, we calculate the gradient differential matrix $\mathbf{D} \in \mathbb{R}^{320\times240\times2}$, a matrix of two-dimensional vectors $\boldsymbol{d}_{i,j}$. We also calculate its Euclidean norm and tangent matrices, $\mathbf{D}_{mod}, \mathbf{D}_{\alpha} \in \mathbb{R}^{320\times240}$, as follows [51]:

$$\boldsymbol{d}_{i,j} = \left(d_{x_{i,j}}, d_{y_{i,j}}\right) = (\, i_{i+1,j} - i_{i-1,j}, i_{i,j+1} - i_{i,j-1})$$

$$\mathrm{d}_{mod_{i,j}} = \|\boldsymbol{d}_{i,j}\| = \sqrt{{d_{x_{i,j}}}^2 + {d_{y_{i,j}}}^2}, \mathrm{d}_{\alpha_{i,j}} = \tan^{-1}(\frac{d_{y_{i,j}}}{d_{x_{i,j}}})$$

A histogram of the values of $\mathbf{D}_{mod}$ and $\mathbf{D}_{\alpha}$ is then calculated in 16x16 pixel blocks. Based on this histogram, a Support Vector Machine determines if the frame contains a face, as described in [51, 71]. We use this implementation because it shows more robustness than other options, such as the Viola and Jones algorithm [328, 329].

If the frame is determined to contain a face, facial features are detected (3). This process consists of determining the most likely position of 68 facial features (points of the eyes, nose and mouth), including those necessary for EAR calculation. For this purpose, we used a Dlib implementation of the algorithm presented in Kazemi et al. [151]. This method is based on a gradient tree regression cascade that iteratively estimates the position of each feature. The procedure works as follows: let $\boldsymbol{x}$ be the (i, j) pixel estimated position of a facial feature in the image, and $\mathbf{S} \in \mathbb{R}^{2\times n} = ({\boldsymbol{x}_1}^T, {\boldsymbol{x}_2}^T, \dots, {\boldsymbol{x}_n}^T)$ be the matrix defining the coordinates of all n facial features, with $\hat{\mathbf{S}}^{(k)}$ being the k-th iteration of the estimation of **S** ($\hat{\mathbf{S}}^{(0)}$ is the average of the training data applied over the image), and reg_k the regression operator, then [151]:

$$\hat{\mathbf{S}}^{(k+1)} = \hat{\mathbf{S}}^{(k)} + reg_k(\mathbf{I}, \hat{\mathbf{S}}^{(k)}), k = 0,1, \dots, K$$

This consists on K iterations, one per regressor, where regressors are trained on a given dataset. Regressors take both the latest estimation $\hat{\mathbf{S}}^{(k)}$ as well as the intensity matrix **I**, as calculated above, into consideration. The last iteration results in the best approximation of the position of all facial features **S**.

The position of the eye pupil is then determined (4). This process is performed using gradient vector angles as described in Timm and Barth [315]. This method takes a 50 pixel region around the geometric center of the EAR points estimated in **S**, and calculates the point near the center of the image where most gradient vectors intersect and pixel intensity is at its highest $\boldsymbol{c}$, as the pupil is the darkest region of the eye. More specifically, it performs the following calculation. Let $\hat{\boldsymbol{c}}$ be the (i, j) coordinates of an eye center candidate, and $\boldsymbol{x}_n$ be the (i, j) coordinates of pixel n of the 50 pixel selection, then:

$$\boldsymbol{c} = \arg\max\left\{\frac{1}{50}\sum_{n=1}^{50} w_n({\boldsymbol{l}_n}^T\boldsymbol{d}_{i,j})^2\right\}, \boldsymbol{l}_n = \frac{\boldsymbol{x}_n - \hat{\boldsymbol{c}}}{\|\boldsymbol{x}_n - \hat{\boldsymbol{c}}\|}$$

Where $\boldsymbol{d}_{i,j}$ is the gradient vector of pixel n, as calculated above, and $w_n \in [0,1]$ is a normalized weight based on pixel intensity $i_{i,j}$. $\hat{\boldsymbol{c}}$ candidates are all points where $w_n > 0.9$, which means that they are particularly dark in comparison with the rest of the image. From all these candidates, the point where the gradients are at its maximum corresponds to the location where most gradients intersect, which is then defined as the eye center.

Finally, if the eye features and a pupil are found, the frame is considered valid and the EAR is calculated (5). Once a continuous EAR time series is produced, blinks can be detected when the EAR is lower than the threshold value of 0.2 [290]. However, the average blinking speed and framerate have to be taken into consideration. A blink takes 290 to 750 ms on average, or 1.33 to 3.45 Hz, and mean blink-rates range from 2 to 50 blinks per minute. The closing time is on average longer than the opening time [279]. Given that our camera framerate is 20 Hz, we found that a frame can be classified as a blink if it is the third of a series of frames with $EAR < 0.20$. *Figure 56* presents a summary of this algorithm.

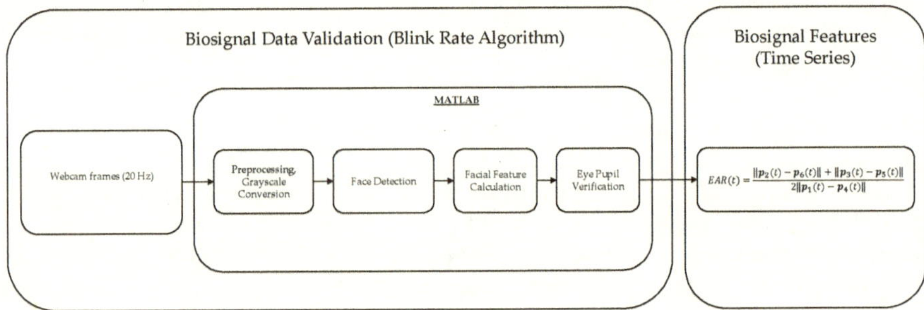

Figure 56: Eye aspect ratio biosignal processing diagram

Evaluation

To evaluate the accuracy of our algorithm, we compare its results with a manual blink count on a series of samples. In this sense, a TP implies a blink that occurred and was detected, a FP is a falsely detected blink, a FN is a non-detected blink, and a TN is a frame in which no blink occurred nor was detected. Most samples are thus TN, which means the specificity is not representative of performance. Thus, for this scenario, we present the results for precision and TP rate (*Table 51*), which is what other authors also present.

A cohort of ten participants watched a five-minute video, sitting at a distance of 50 cm from a computer screen with a maximum angle between the face and screen of 35 degrees. There were no inclusion or exclusion criteria. Users were not aware that the blink-rate was being calculated. In addition to this database, we tested our algorithm in two publicly available databases: TALK [306] and Eyeblink8 [62]. In *Table 30*, we present the results of our algorithm and other available options in these databases. We include results for participant-weighted averages, in which the results are normalized by the number of participants in each database. The complete results are provided in *Appendix G, Table 67* and *Table 68*. Information about these databases, such as framerate and resolutions, is also provided in *Appendix G, Table 70*.

As detailed in *Table 30,* results indicate that our algorithm has better precision results (participant-weighted average of 0.84) than TP rate results (participant-weighted average of 0.73). This implies that our algorithm rarely detects false blinks, but misses a number of actual blinks. More specifically, on average, one in every four blinks was not detected. Interestingly, our algorithm performed worse than Soukupová et al. [290] in the database Eyeblink8. We suspect this is highly dependent on how well-adjusted the EAR threshold is to the specific database in which the evaluation is performed. For example, our algorithm performed very well in the TALK database and our own database, which is the one with the largest cohort. Based on these results, we conclude that although the EAR is a good parameter to detect blinks, EAR-based blink detection requires a more sophisticated detection method than a threshold. Nevertheless, the first step to improve these results would be to collect a larger database of users and blinks with which to base any assumptions on potential improvements over threshold-based calculations. In any case, our results support the idea of using a web camera and a simple blink-rate detection algorithm to monitor the blink-rate of PD patients in the background while they are interacting with an exergame. In addition, an increased framerate would allow us not only to detect blinks, but also to calculate parameters related to eye opening and closing speed during blinking, based on EAR differentials. These could potentially discriminate severity of bradykinesia and ON-OFF periods in PD, in a similar fashion to the parameters with extracts from the Leap Motion sensor in *Chapter 6*.

Reference	Drutarovsky et al. [62]	Lee et al. [186]	Divjak et al. [58]	Soukupová et al. [290]	Our algorithm
TALK [306], precision	0.92	0.83	0.83		0.93
TALK [306], TP rate	0.97	0.91			0.8
Eyeblink8 [62], precision	0.79			0.94	0.62
Eyeblink8 [62], TP rate	0.85			0.96	0.68
Our Database, precision					0.93
Our database, TP rate					0.75
Participant-weighted average, precision	0.82	0.83	0.83	0.94	0.84
Participant-weighted average, TP rate	0.87	0.91		0.96	0.73

Table 30: Blink-rate algorithm results when using other author's databases

8. Alternative Game-based Interventions

In *Chapter 5* and *Chapter 6,* two proofs of concept of exergame-based clinical decision support systems are presented. As a secondary goal in this book, we explored alternative game-based approaches other than exergames to design clinical decision support systems to monitor PD symptoms. We identified two possible alternatives, which we described in the section *Other Game-based Interventions* of *Chapter 3*. As part of this book, we explored the possibility of using BCIs as well as VR-based games. We designed a BCI system to control a game with a different number of possible commands, and tested the system exploring how classification accuracy decreases as the number of possible commands increases. This study was published in [89]. Our preliminary results suggest that the features we used, captured with surface electroencephalography, did not allow us to control a serious game with more than two commands with sufficient accuracy. Concerning VR, we developed a dual-tasking block-breaking VR game, controlled with the Leap Motion sensor, entitled Brix [19]. Unfortunately, early in our design, we noticed many users experienced motion sickness in VR, commonly known as cybersickness. For this reason, we discarded the use of VR as a main component of this book. However, we conducted a number of studies into cybersickness, its causes and potential solutions for future work. First, we performed a systematic review and meta-analysis of the possible causes of cybersickness, and how different devices and locomotion techniques affect it [34]. We found that heart-rate variability is a potential indicator of cybersickness [96], and developed a clinical decision support system to detect it [95]. As a possible solution, we considered polynomial extrapolation to more accurately predict head movements and positions [98]. Experimental details of these studies are also provided in *Appendix H.*

8.1. Brain-Computer Interfaces

A BCI is a system capable of interpreting brain activity directly to control a computer application. Usually, this is achieved with surface electroencephalography. There are several BCI-controlled serious games available, for example the football game "Brain Arena" [26], or the one presented in [49], in which the player controls a spaceship and dodges asteroids. Classification accuracies vary greatly, depending among others on the number of possible commands. For example, using two commands usually shows accuracies of 80% or more, while [49] reports an accuracy of approximately 60% when four possible commands are used. In our opinion, playing a game in which commands are only correctly registered 60% of the time is not feasible. In general, BCIs show great promise, not only for PD but in many other domains [220]. This inspired us to analyze how accuracy decreases in a BCI controlled game as the number of commands increases using recent advances in BCI classification [191]. A summary of accuracies depending on the number of commands for different available BCI-controlled games from the literature is presented in *Table 31.*

When using surface electroencephalography to control an application, the goal is to detect changes in the signals caused by an external stimulus, for example an image. These alterations are called event-related potentials. A very typical event-related potential is a peak detected 250 to 500 ms after the stimulus, known as P300 [323]. A simple binary classification could thus be performed based on the presence, or absence, of a P300. When attempting to classify more than two possibilities, we hypothesized there would be differences in the event-related potentials of different electrodes, particularly on the motor cortex (*Figure 57*, nodes C5 to C6). In a preliminary analysis, we did observe that when the participant thinks of different limbs, the amplitudes of these potentials change slightly.

For example, when thinking about moving the left arm, the amplitude of P300 in sensor C2 was higher. These differences suggest that a limb-based classification could be feasible. We decided to evaluate this hypothesis.

Number of commands	Accuracy (maximum, %)	Accuracy (average, %)	Reference
Two (increase, decrease in focus)	65	69	[193]
Two (yes, no)	85	79	[78]
Two (left, right)	89	81	[178]
Two (left, right)	76	74	[26]
Two (left, right)/four (foot, tongue)	85/69	80/60	[49]

Table 31: Effect of the number of possible commands on classification accuracy in BCIs

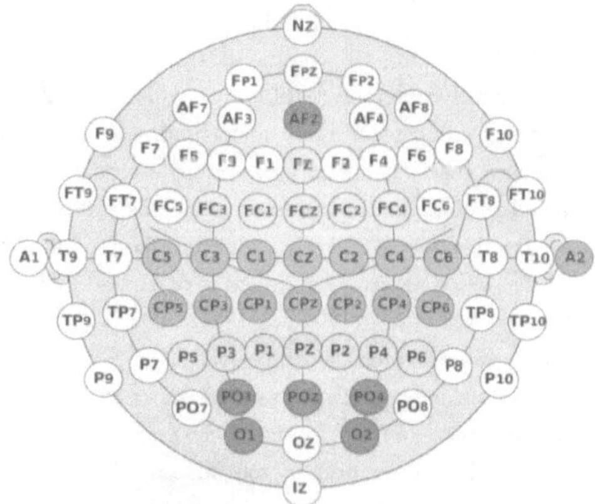

Figure 57: 10-20 electrode placement to acquire the electroencephalographic signal [60]

In order to acquire the electroencephalographic signal, we used the USBAmp biosignal amplifier with a 32 unipolar electrode cap and the 10-20 electrode placement system [262] and a sampling frequency of 200 Hz. The data was filtered with a 50 Hz notch filter and a 0.5-60 Hz 5th order bandpass filter. To remove outliers, we considered two options: the standard deviation method described in [190] and a moving average filter with a window of 0.25 seconds [77].

To test the system, we conceived a game that aimed at classifying eight different commands, that is, seven commands and a neutral state. We created a climbing game in which the player may command movements in each of their limbs (left arm, right arm, left leg, right leg), a combination of two of them (both arms, both legs) and an extra action (eating a fly when it's visible in screen). For each step, the direction required to progress is visually depicted. The game is programmed so that in order to progress, all actions have to be used. This means that, for example, at a certain point during the climb, it is only possible to proceed by moving the left arm, or the right leg. We did this to ensure that all possible commands had to be used in each scenario. A system diagram is presented in *Figure 58*.

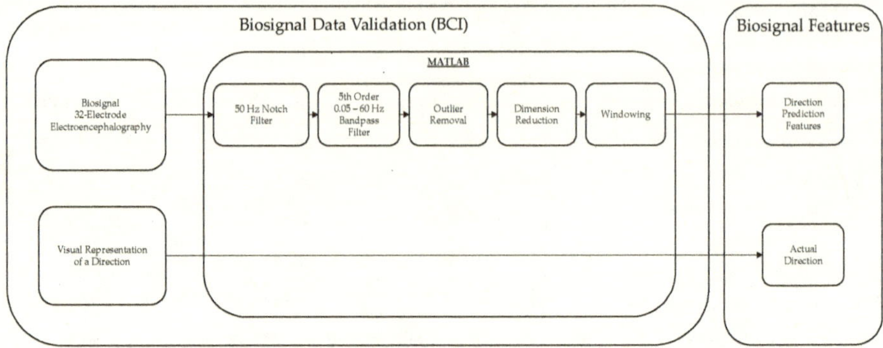

Figure 58: Electroencephalographic biosignal processing diagram

To evaluate the accuracy of our system, we compared the visually depicted actions with BCI predictions. We collected data from five users. five-fold cross validation was used to classify the data. The recording was performed using a two-second relaxation phase and a five-second recording section. During the recording section, an image was visually presented on the screen that suggested the user which action to think about (which limb to move). Each class was presented five times, following a random pattern. For feature extraction, we used the wavelet transform method [8] as well as FFT-based frequency domain analysis. A list of the features employed is presented in *Table 32*.

After acquiring our data, and based on classification accuracy, we performed changes in data processing. We found that an outlier detection system based on standard deviation delivered slightly better performance than a moving average filter. With this system, sensor values are removed if their value exceeds 2.8 times the standard deviation of the surrounding five frames. We found that dimension reduction using t-distributed stochastic neighbor embedding, as suggested in [191], did not increase accuracy. We also studied how analyzing different sample lengths after presenting the stimulus affects the accuracy. We considered possible lengths of 0.5, 1, 2 and 4 seconds. We found there is little difference between employing 2 and 4 seconds, but using shorter lengths significantly decreased accuracy. Focusing classification to a subset of electrodes, for example the motor cortex, did not increase accuracy.

The outcomes of the analysis suggest that static energy features performed best on average. A support vector machine using a poly-kernel was the best classification method, achieving a maximum accuracy of 80% with two possible commands (both hands and both legs, plus the neutral state). However, average accuracy was not sufficiently high to elicit claims of validity. In general, we found large interindividual differences in accuracy. A summary of our classification results is presented in *Table 33*.

Feature	Description	Reference
E_{R_i}	Daubechies 4 wavelet transformation, relative energy of each of the 5 time series (d_1 to d_4 and a_5) with a sample length of n frames, divided by total energy. Five features per electrode. Based on [8]	$E_{D_i} = \sum_{j=1}^{n} d_{i,j}^2, i = 1,2,3,4, E_A = \sum_{j=1}^{n} a_{5,j}^2,$ $E_{R_i} = \frac{E_{D_i}}{\sum_{j=1}^{4} E_{D_j} + E_A}, i = 1,2,3,4$ $E_{R_5} = \frac{E_A}{\sum_{j=1}^{4} E_{D_j} + E_A}$
$Diff_{Avg\,i,k}$	Daubechies 4 mean value of wavelets 2 and 3, difference between electrode k and average value across all m electrodes. Two features per electrode. Based on [191]	$\bar{d}_{i,k} = \frac{\sum_{j=1}^{n} d_{i,j}}{n}, i = 2,3, k = 1, \dots, m$ $Diff_{Avg\,i,k} = \bar{d}_{i,k} - \frac{\sum_{l=1,l \neq k}^{m} \bar{d}_{i,l}}{m-1}, i = 2,3, k = 1, \dots, m$
$Diff_{Energy\,i,k}$	Daubechies 4 mean energy of wavelets 2 and 3, difference between electrode k and average value across all m electrodes. Two features per electrode. Based on [191]	$\bar{E}_{i,k} = \frac{\sum_{j=1}^{n} d_{i,j}^2}{n}, i = 2,3, k = 1, \dots, m$ $Diff_{Energy\,i,k} = \bar{E}_{i,k} - \frac{\sum_{l=1,l \neq k}^{m} \bar{E}_{i,l}}{m-1}, i = 2,3, k = 1, \dots, m$
$Diff_{Std\,i,k}$	Daubechies 4 standard deviation of wavelets 2 and 3, difference between electrode k and average value across all m electrodes. Two features per electrode. Based on [191]	$\bar{S}_{i,k} = \sqrt{\frac{\sum_{j=1}^{n}(d_{i,j} - \bar{d}_{i,k})^2}{n-1}}, i = 2,3, k = 1, \dots, m$ $Diff_{Std\,i,k} = \bar{S}_{i,k} - \frac{\sum_{l=1,l \neq k}^{m} \bar{S}_{i,l}}{m-1}, i = 2,3, k = 1, \dots, m$
$Energy_{Alpha}$, $Energy_{Beta}$, $Energy_{Gamma}$	Total energy of the alpha (7-13 Hz), beta (13-39 Hz), gamma waves (>40 Hz) and residual energy	See Table 21, $Energy_{Total}$

Table 32: BCI system preliminary features

Number of commands (plus neutral state)	Accuracy (maximum, %)	Accuracy (average, %)
Two	80%	56%
Three	74%	44%
Four	50%	31%
Five	45%	29%

Table 33: BCI system classification preliminary results

Although a BCI seemed a viable approach to assess cognitive skills in principle, particularly in PD patients with severe motor symptoms, due to these accuracy results, we decided not to consider BCI games as a potential scenario for our system.

8.2. Virtual Reality

As we discussed in the section *Other Game-based Interventions* of *Chapter 3*, VR has shown great potential in rehabilitation scenarios. It seems to have as positive an impact as traditional exergames [43, 205], while increasing immersion and fun [35, 36]. In the initial steps of this book, we designed a dual-tasking VR game prototype entitled Brix [19] (*Figure 59*), as a block-breaking VR game that is controlled with physical hand movements with the Leap Motion sensor.

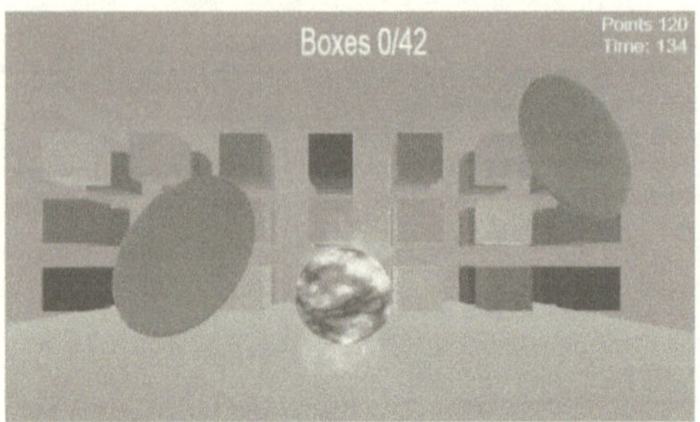

Figure 59: Block-breaking VR game Brix. The disks follow the hand position and their diameter is controlled by opening and closing the fist

While designing Brix, we noticed most participants experienced motion sickness a few minutes after starting to play. This phenomenon, also known as cybersickness, is widely reported in VR [47, 162, 265, 266, 271, 294]. Even if our scenario did barely include physical movements, cybersickness was still present. For this reason, we discarded the use of VR as one of the main application scenarios in this book. However, this provided us with an additional research field: although cybersickness is not a disease, it does cause a physiological response [96]. In addition, cybersickness is currently evaluated by a questionnaire, named Simulator Sickness Questionnaire (SSQ) [154]. As is the case with the UPDRS test, its potential subjectivity has been discussed [343]. In theory, an implementation of the concept described in *Chapter 4* to detect cybersickness could be feasible, and provide objective criteria to determine the presence of cybersickness . If feasible, it could be used to determine the eligibility of a patient for VR-based rehabilitation, if their cybersickness susceptibility is sufficiently low. In this section, we present our research towards a clinical decision support system designed to detect cybersickness.

In order to study how cybersickness affects players in modern VR devices, we conducted a systematic review, published in [34]. We identified numerous potential factors that influence cybersickness, which we summarize in *Appendix H, Table 71*. We observed that modern VR systems, such as the HTC Vive, use teleportation-based locomotion, where the user points at a visible position and they are teleported there without a virtual movement taking place. This locomotion method causes significantly less cybersickness than virtual translational movements. Recent literature suggests that possible solutions to cybersickness are adding a virtual nose [338] or restricting VR locomotion to teleportation [44]. In [98, 337], we explored the possibility of reducing the discrepancy between virtual and physical movements by interpolating head angular positions by using linear extrapolation combined with a Savitzky-Golay filter. We found that low prediction errors (e.g., 0.04 arc degrees for typical VR gameplay) can be achieved when extrapolating up to 13 ms. This, however, would only partially remove one of the many causes of cybersickness. User adaptation seems to be the best strategy at the moment [138]. Thus, we considered the possibility of designing a system that can detect cybersickness instead.

The gold standard to evaluate the presence of cybersickness is the SSQ [154]. It presents questions on a series of symptoms commonly associated with cybersickness, administered before and after the VR experience. In the questionnaire, users are asked about the severity of these symptoms giving each of them a score ranging from zero (no symptoms) to three (severe symptoms). The questionnaire then provides four scores as a result, one for each domain of cybersickness (nausea, oculomotor, disorientation) and a global score. The VR experience can then be categorized based on the scores of several users into negligible cybersickness (total score lower than 5), minimal (5 to 10), significant (10 to 15), concerning (15 to 20) and bad (greater than 20). When comparing modern VR to the traditional flight simulators the SSQ was designed for, it is typical for cybersickness to present higher scores in disorientation [162, 179, 199, 294, 296] and lower scores in oculomotor symptoms and nausea [274, 296]. Thus, the symptomatologic profile of cybersickness significantly differs from other VR options, such as immersive flight simulators [271, 296].

An alternative to using the SSQ is to explore the physiological response to cybersickness. In [96], we conducted a preliminary study exploring how cybersickness affects the heart-rate variability. In this study, we measured the 2-lead ECG of 13 users (median age 22, two females) while they played the game QuakeVR [260] using an Oculus Rift Developer Kit 2 for 15 minutes. We calculated the SSQ scores, the mean values of N-N intervals, and the standard deviation of N-N intervals. We observed statistically significant differences (p=0.02) between the participants that did and did not suffer cybersickness, as measured by the SSQ scores. We also calculated the Pearson correlation between these two N-N interval features and the SSQ scores, but did not find particularly high correlations. The results of this study are provided in *Appendix H, Table 73* and *Table 74*.

In our systematic review, we also studied other recent publications exploring the physiological response to cybersickness. A summary of these studies is presented in *Appendix H, Table 72*. More recent studies suggest that the reaction most correlated with cybersickness is an increase in galvanic skin response, which refers to changes in sweat gland activity. Six studies report statistical significance [55, 95, 100, 101, 160, 162]. On the contrary, although VR does impact heart-rate and heart-rate variability, the direction in which this variation is experienced (tachycardia or bradycardia) is largely an interindividual difference, and thus it does not seem to be a good criterion to predict cybersickness by itself. However, it may be used in combination with other data sources. After conducting this research, we believed it was feasible to design a clinical decision support system to diagnose cybersickness, because in our preliminary study [96] and our systematic review [34], there was significant evidence of a physiological, measurable response to cybersickness.

To achieve this goal, we developed a virtual reality game called VRFlight (*Figure 60*), that submits the player to lateral movements and rotations. In it, the player controls a plane with a traditional console controller, while experiencing the environment in VR. The player is encouraged to move the plane to collect coins on their path. As the player's perspective is fixed to the plane, any movement performed by it is also experienced by the player, but it is not correlated to a real physical movement. However, a player can orient their head freely. This scenario is known to cause significant cybersickness. The game was developed in Unity3D [321] using iTween [21].

The game is composed of four levels, and divided into two similar scenarios. In one scenario, the plane moves only laterally, and in the other scenario the plane only performs barrel rolls. This was done to ensure a more diverse profile of cybersickness was created. First, a 3.5-minute tutorial is used as an introduction to the VR experience, and to provide a baseline with which to compare scenarios with more movement. During this tutorial, the plane moves in a straight line and the player does not perform any movement at the beginning. After three minutes, the player is asked to perform a single movement, either a lateral movement or a rotation. Afterwards, the game contains three more levels:

- Level 1 (3 minutes), in which the plane follows a straight line.
- Level 2 (3.5 minutes) in which the plain moves upwards and downwards, then left and right.
- Level 3 (3 minutes) in which the planes moves in all directions and environmental elements (tunnels, trees) are present.

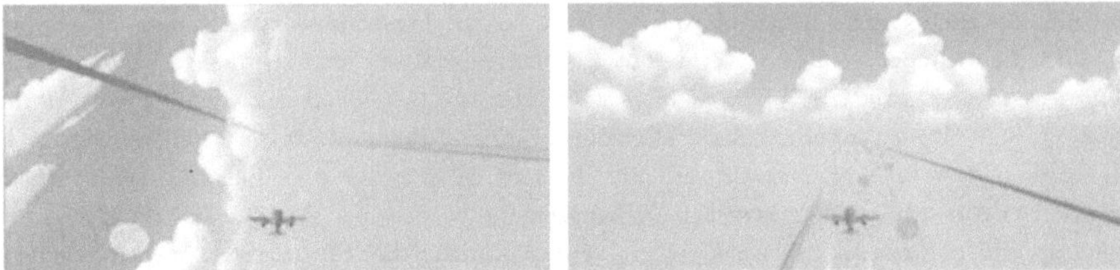

Figure 60: VRFlight game [95]

We evaluate the accuracy of this clinical decision support system by comparing it with the results of the SSQ, collected directly before and directly after the VR experience. In this evaluation, we collect data from VRFlight (game data), from the VR device (interaction data), as well as biosignals. A cohort of 66 participants were randomly assigned to the rotation or the lateral movement group. While the game was running, the following biosignals were captured: two-lead ECG (*Figure 50)*, respiratory effort, electrooculography, and galvanic skin response. The respiratory effort was measured with a chest expansion strap to derive the respiratory rate. Electrooculography was captured using gel electrodes, as depicted in *Figure 61*. Finally, galvanic skin response was measured using two finger electrodes, as a measure of sweat gland activity. All signals were captured using a USBAmp biosignal amplifier, with a sampling rate of 200 Hz and a 50 Hz notch filter. We used cubic spline interpolation to synchronize data sources. A diagram summarizing processing is presented in *Figure 63*.

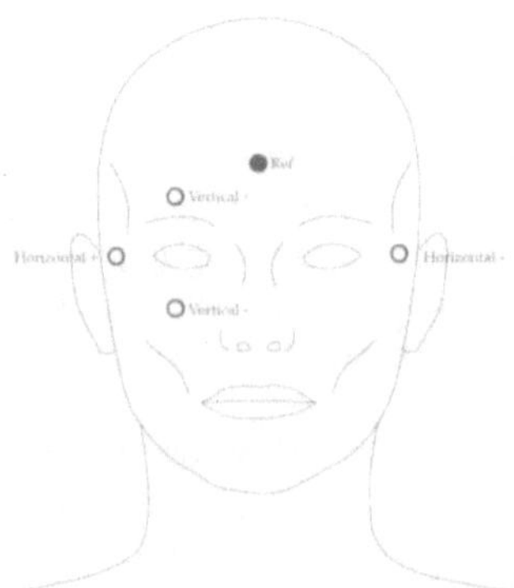

Figure 61: Electrode placement to acquire the electrooculographic signal. Courtesy of [195]

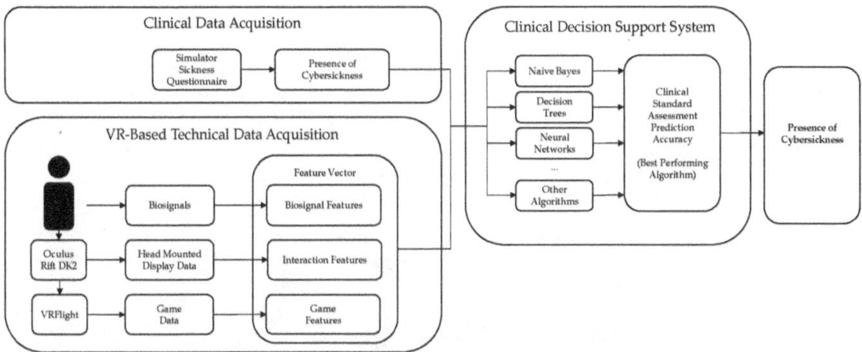

Figure 62: VR-based clinical decision support system to assess cybersickness. System diagram

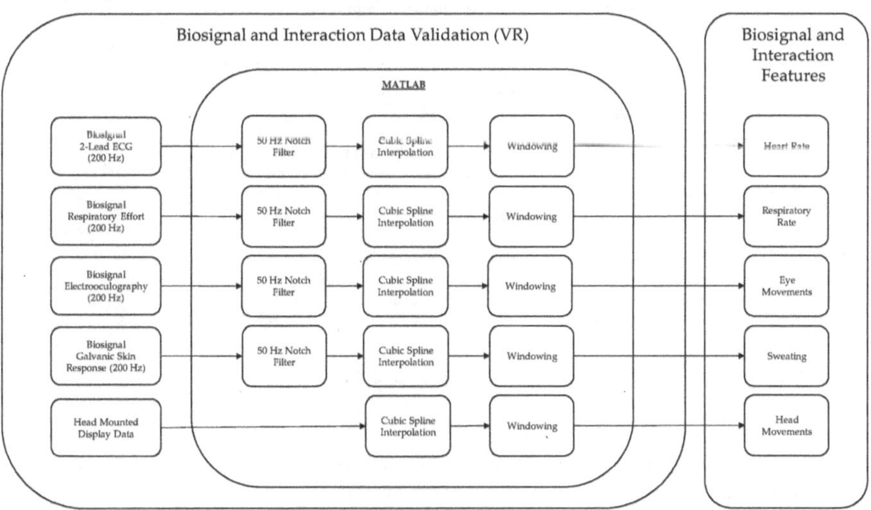

Figure 63: VR system biosignal and interaction data processing diagram

We obtained the best results using a K-Nearest Neighbours algorithm, with preliminary results presented in *Table 35*. The maximum achieved accuracy of 58% does not elicit the claim that the proposed method is capable of accurately estimating the severity of the experienced VR sickness. Increasing epoch length to 60 seconds did not increase accuracy. In general, the system tends to predict worse cybersickness scores than the ones measured by the SSQ. We observed that game data, and sensor data (particularly head movements) performed better than biosignals. When considering features individually, the accuracies of most features is similar and around 45%. Head acceleration provided the best individual results (49%) followed by plane speed (47%), position (46%) and angular acceleration (40%). This supports the hypothesis that at least certain biosignals do not relate to the physiological response to cybersickness.

Feature	Description	Reference
HR_{Avg}	Heart-rate per 30-second epoch, using a heartbeat detection algorithm as described in *Chapter 7* to calculate the number of heartbeats $n_{Heartbeats}$. One feature per epoch.	$2\ n_{Heartbeats}$
RR_{Avg}	Average respiratory rate per 30-second epoch, using the same peak detection algorithm as above to obtain the number of breaths $n_{Breaths}$. One feature per epoch	$2\ n_{Breaths}$
$EOG_{Vert_{Avg}}$	Average vertical electrooculography value per 30-second epoch, where $EOG_{Vert}(t)$ is the time series, with n frames per epoch. One feature per epoch	$\frac{\sum_{t=1}^{n} EOG_{Vert}(t)}{n}$
$EOG_{Horz_{Avg}}$	Average horizontal electrooculography value per 30-second epoch, where $EOG_{Horz}(t)$ is the time series, with n frames per epoch. One feature per epoch	$\frac{\sum_{t=1}^{n} EOG_{Horz}(t)}{n}$
GSR_{Avg}	Average galvanic skin response value per 30-second epoch, where $GSR(t)$ is the time series, with n frames per epoch. One feature per epoch	$\frac{\sum_{t=1}^{n} GSR(t)}{n}$
$Head_{Pos_{Linear}}$, $Head_{Speed_{Linear}}$, $Head_{Acc_{Linear}}$	Linear position, speed and acceleration of the head obtained from the head-mounted display. Average value per 30-second epoch, three-dimensional (x, y, z). Calculation provided as example for $Head_{Pos_{Linear}}$, with n frames per epoch. Nine features per epoch.	$\frac{\sum_{t=1}^{n} Head_{Pos_{Linear}}(t)}{n}$
$Head_{Pos_{Angular}}$, $Head_{Speed_{Angular}}$, $Head_{Acc_{Angular}}$	Angular position, speed and acceleration of the head obtained from the head-mounted display. Average value per 30-second epoch, three-dimensional $(pitch, yaw, roll)$. Calculation provided as example for $Head_{Pos_{Angular}}$, with n frames per epoch. Nine features per epoch	$\frac{\sum_{t=1}^{n} Head_{Pos_{Angular}}(t)}{n}$
$Plane_{Pos}$, $Plane_{Speed}$, $Plane_{Acc}$	Position, speed and acceleration of the plane (in respect to the central position). Average value per 30-second epoch. Linear (x, y, z) values in the lateral movement version, angular $(pitch, yaw, roll)$ values in the rotation version. Calculation provided as example for $Plane_{Pos}$, with n frames per epoch. Nine features per epoch	$\frac{\sum_{t=1}^{n} Plane_{Pos}(t)}{n}$
$Controller_{Inputs}$	Number of controller inputs per 30-second epoch. One feature per epoch	
$N_{Objects}$	Total number of visible objects per 30-second epoch. One feature per epoch	
$N_{Collisions}$	Total number of collisions (including coins) per 30-second epoch. One feature per epoch	

Table 34: Cybersickness system preliminary features

Classification Accuracy	Total	Nausea	Oculomotor	Disorientation
Per Playthrough	58%	42%	50%	44%
Per Level	41%	35%	45%	39%

Table 35: Cybersickness susceptibility system classification preliminary results

9. Summary, Conclusions and Future Work

PD is a neurodegenerative disease that requires constant monitoring to adjust medication, assess risks and monitor its progress. It also presents large interindividual differences. Combined with the subjectivity of current PD monitoring methods, such as the UPDRS scale, this implies the need for more objective symptom assessment methods. In this book, we propose the use of exergame-based clinical decision support systems to monitor symptoms of PD. This approach presents several advantages. First, it provides neurologists with more objective information with which to perform medical decisions. Second, it provides an engaging environment for patients to provide clinically meaningful data. In this chapter, we summarize our work, highlight our main contributions, discuss our conclusions, and provide guidelines for potential future research.

9.1. Summary of the book

In *Chapter 1,* we identify two main challenges when implementing exergame-based clinical decision support systems for PD. The first challenge is to design sensor-based environments that can be used to monitor a certain symptom. This environment has to be designed on a case-by-case basis. The chosen sensor, or combination of sensors, must simultaneously provide clinically meaningful data on the symptom in question and be usable as a control device for an exergame. The second challenge is to design an exergame, controlled by this sensor, that is attractive and engaging for the target population. If the data acquisition requires the participants to perform certain movements, such as those performed in the UPDRS test, the exergame must incorporate these movements as well. In this book, we address these challenges by designing two exergame-based clinical decision support systems. The first system assesses balance and the risk of falling, and the second system assesses hand tremor and bradykinesia (slow movements).

In *Chapter 2,* we briefly present the foundations for our model design: exergames, patient monitoring, and clinical decision support systems. Furthermore, in *Chapter 3,* we present two systematic reviews on possible sensors to implement our model, and the state of the art of exergame-based rehabilitation interventions in PD. Based on these results, we decided to use the Wii Balance Board to assess balance and the risk of falling, and the Leap Motion sensor to assess hand tremor and bradykinesia. In both cases, there are alternative sensors that could have been employed instead. For example, the Microsoft Kinect can be used to assess balance, but we found that when implementing exergames for rehabilitation the Wii Balance Board shows better results in clinical trials. Conversely, it is also possible to assess tremor using smartwatches. However, we intended to design systems in which patients do not have to wear any device themselves, and thus avoided wearables. Our reviews also indicate that exergame-based interventions in PD can be as effective as traditional rehabilitation, in some cases even providing better results. An additional advantage of this approach is that combining cognitive and motor tasks, known as dual-tasking, further improves rehabilitation results. However, statistically significant results are still scarce.

Contributions

In this book, we define and address two main goals and two secondary goals. Our two main goals are to design, implement, and validate a clinical decision support system to assess balance and a clinical decision support system to assess hand tremor and bradykinesia. These goals are defined as two proofs of concept of the model presented in *Chapter 4.* Our two secondary goals are to explore additional biosignals that could be acquired while the PD patient plays the exergame, and to study alternative game-based approaches other than exergames to access further valuable data.

In *Chapter 4,* we present our model for an exergame-based clinical decision support system designed to assess a symptom of PD. This model collects data from the exergame, from the sensor implemented to interact with the game, and from additional biosignal modules. These data are converted into a series of features employed by a clinical decision support system trained with medical information from the patient to provide clinically meaningful data. The medical partners can use these data as an additional source of information to perform medical decisions.

In *Chapter 5,* we design, implement, and validate the model presented in *Chapter 4* to design a clinical decision support system to assess balance. In this chapter, we present a novel interaction sensor, the Extended Balance Board, designed as an array of Wii Balance Boards. This sensor has the advantage of providing a larger surface of sensors, thus being capable of assessing the balance while standing and walking. We also tested an alternative system that collected data from additional sources, namely electromyography and sensor accelerometers. However, a preliminary study did not suggest that this system had an advantage over the Extended Balance Board. We also present PDDanceCity, an exergame that combines a cognitive and motor task, and that can provide data related to balance and cognition. We evaluate this system's capability to detect players with an age- and sex-adjusted increased risk of falling, and to perform a general prediction without player-specific information. For this purpose, we design a clinical decision support system that attempts to predict the result of the 30-Second-Sit-To-Stand Test, based on data obtained from PDDanceCity and the Extended Balance Board. We tested this system with a cohort of 16 participants (7 with balance affections), and considered two potential scenarios: predicting the result without and with player-specific information (age and sex). In both cases, we achieved prediction accuracies of over 90%, highlighting how this system can accurately detect players that show balance problems while standing and walking. Including age and sex as classification features, in this case predicting an age- and sex-adjusted risk of falling, provided slightly better results (95%). We also performed an acceptance test of PDDanceCity with the target population, with positive results. 80% of participants found the game to be user-friendly and fun, while only 66% would play it from home if it were available. We believe this is due to the interaction between the Extended Balance Board and PDDanceCity, which shows some potential for improvement. We also believe that PDDanceCity would see benefit in a more immersive environment.

In *Chapter 6*, we design, implement, and validate the model presented in *Chapter 4* to design a clinical decision support system to assess hand tremor and bradykinesia. For this purpose, we conceived a digitalized version of the UPDRS tasks designed to monitor these symptoms (UPDRS tasks 3.4 to 3.6, 3.15 and 3.16). We call this software Parkinson Assessment with Leap Motion (PALM). In PALM, we extract features related to tremor amplitude and frequency, as well as features related to how the patient performs the UPDRS tasks. These features are based on the evaluation criteria described in the UPDRS guidelines. We also design a kinetic signal processing system that filters and crops the data obtained from the Leap Motion sensor. We then present PDPuzzleTable, an exergame that combines a cognitive and motor task, and can provide data related to cognition, as well as the data we obtain with PALM. In this chapter, we employ data from five PD patients and five healthy controls to evaluate the capability of a clinical decision support system to discriminate the data from the PD patients and the controls. We consider two separate evaluation scenarios: classification based on resting tremor features, and based on kinetic tasks. Classification results are in both cases excellent, with accuracies at or close to 95%. All misclassified samples belonged to a PD patient who had a very recent diagnosis and was under medication at the time of data acquisition. Unfortunately, we did not see any characteristics in this patient's data that helped us further improve the classification. Although the small sample size did not allow us to achieve statistical significance in all scenarios, effect sizes in most cases indicate the described features could also be able to predict UPDRS scores in the future. This sample size does not allow us to estimate if our approach is better than the best performing methods in the related work ([330] for resting tremor, see *Table 3* and [74] for bradykinesia, see *Table 4*), but our results are comparable in accuracy and our new features, described in *Table 21* and *Table 22 do* show statistical significance and large effect sizes. We conclude this chapter with an acceptance test of PDPuzzleTable. 92% of participants found the game to be fun, and its difficulty adjustment settings to be adequate. However, as the difficulty increases and we remove the mechanisms we implemented to ease sensor interaction, player performance drops significantly. This suggests that the learning effect of the interaction with a Leap Motion sensor has to be taken into consideration when using PDPuzzleTable to assess cognition, particularly at higher difficulty levels. Nevertheless, this learning effect is also a potential measure of cognition.

In *Chapter 7,* we discuss potential biosignal modules that can be employed as part of any exergame-based clinical decision support system. These modules can be used to monitor additional symptoms of PD, or to improve system accuracy with sensor fusion. We provide one example of each of these modules, a heart-rate variability acquisition system based on PPG, and a blink-rate measurement system on the example of a webcam. PD has been shown to affect heart-rate variability, and dyskinesia affects the blink-rate as well as hand dexterity. The heart-rate variability system extracts frames from a smartphone camera, and then uses a novel processing method to calculate the time interval between heartbeats. The blink-rate estimation algorithm is based on assessing dimensional changes of different points of interest of the eye to detect blinks. We test both systems with a gold standard: ECG for our PPG algorithm, and blink count for the blink-rate measurement system. Results suggest our heart-rate variability measurement system has excellent accuracy when timing heartbeats in comparison with electrocardiography. Our PPG signal processing method lowers the absolute error to a third of an unfiltered approach, down to an average absolute error of 9.23 ms. In addition to smartphones, this algorithm could also potentially be used using other cameras, such as webcams [241], while the users play PDDanceCity or PDPuzzleTable. Our blink-rate detection algorithm shows positive preliminary results, but fails to detect one in every four blinks. In the future, a larger sample should be acquired to determine potential changes to signal processing that could improve these results.

Finally, in *Chapter 8,* we discuss two potential game-based approaches alternative to exergames that we explored but discarded. BCIs seem to have potential to help PD patients who are receiving deep brain stimulation or to assess cognition. However, in a preliminary analysis, we were unable to design a game that is controlled with a BCI and permits more control than binary choices with sufficient accuracy. We also explored the possibility of implementing VR exergames, since this would increase immersion and engagement. We found that motion sickness in VR, also called cybersickness, is a significant issue that impedes a more pervasive implementation of VR. We conducted a systematic review on cybersickness, and discussed possible ways of detecting it based on its physiological response. This led us to design a clinical decision support system that could potentially detect cybersickness. Our preliminary results indicate this approach is feasible, but our analysis shows potential for improvement.

9.2. Conclusions and Limitations

In this book, we provide a model for an exergame-based clinical decision support system. We implement this model in two scenarios that monitor PD symptoms: one to monitor balance and the risk of falling it implies, and one to monitor hand tremors and dyskinesias. In both cases, our classification results show the ability of our model to monitor PD symptoms and provide caregivers with clinically meaningful data. Moreover, this system could be implemented in a home scenario, providing caregivers with a continuous stream of information and reducing the need for frequent clinic visits. We also provide examples on additional systems that could run in the background and acquire more information from PD patients, either improving prediction accuracy using sensor fusion, or providing information on additional symptoms. We also explore the possibility of using alternative game-based interventions with BCIs and VR.

Although preliminary classification results are positive, our work presents some limitations. First and foremost, adjustments requested by the ethics committee and the outbreak of the COVID-19 pandemic meant we had to adjust most of our evaluation plans. Thus, our evaluations are done with healthy elderly patients in *Chapter 5*, and with a cohort of five PD participants and five healthy controls in *Chapter 6*. Despite the good results, this implied that statistical power was, in some scenarios, lower than expected. The low sample size of *Chapter 6* meant we could not perform an evaluation on whether the features extracted in PALM can form a basis to predict UPDRS scores. In the case of PALM, our system shows difficulties to detect PD patients that have been diagnosed recently. Future studies attempting to objectively determine hand tremors in PD should consider ensuring a number of PD patients with a recent diagnosis are included. The potential of PALM to discriminate PD from other hand tremor sources, such as essential tremor, could also be explored.

The main goal of our clinical decision support systems is to predict a certain clinical outcome, or clinical evaluation system, based on data extracted from the game, from the interactions, and from other sources. However, there is no single clinical test that is used exclusively in any domain of PD, and a patient can provide different results with different clinical assessment methods. For example, balance can also be evaluated with the Berg Balance Scale, the 10-Meter-Walk Test, or the Tinetti Balance Scale. PD symptoms are also commonly evaluated with the Hoehn and Yahr Scale. In order to predict all these outcomes, it is necessary to provide as much clinical data from the patient as possible, which is not always available. Also, the feasibility of the clinical decision support system to accurately predict this outcome directly depends on the choice of sensor and game. The sensor must acquire data that is related to the symptom, and the game must ensure that the patient performs the same task as in the clinical assessment in question. This means that sensor- and game combinations must be specifically designed for each symptom or disease, and any claims of validity can only be performed on a case-by-case basis.

Finally, although the results of the presented systems are positive, as discussed in *Appendix A*, PD is polysymptomatic, and many PD symptoms can still not be remotely monitored. Nevertheless, these positive results should encourage researchers to expand the presented concept into other scenarios.

In conclusion, we believe the objective, quantifiable results presented in this book indicate that the model discussed in *Chapter 4* is feasible and that the implementations described in *Chapter 5* and *Chapter 6* are functional.

www.ingramcontent.com/pod-product-compliance
Lightning Source LLC
LaVergne TN
LVHW041127150826
845673LV00007B/2203